Ride and Shine

How to Become a Successful Indoor Cycling (or Group Exercise) Instructor

Izabela Ruprik

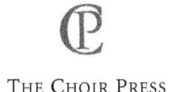

THE CHOIR PRESS

Copyright © 2020 Izabela Ruprik

All rights reserved. No part of this publication may be reproduced or transmitted in any form or by any means, electronic or mechanical including photocopying, recording or any information storage or retrieval system, without prior permission in writing from the publishers.

The right of Izabela Ruprik to be identified as the author of this work has been asserted by her in accordance with the Copyright, Designs and Patents Act 1988

First published in the United Kingdom in 2020 by
The Choir Press

ISBN 978-1-78963-100-5

The author and publisher strongly recommend that you consult with your doctor before beginning any exercise program. You should be in good physical condition and be able to participate in the exercise. The author and publisher are not licensed medical care providers and have no expertise in diagnosing, examining, or treating medical conditions of any kind, or in determining the effect of any specific exercise on a medical condition.

Foreword

They say who needs enemies when you have friends who tell you to proactively pursue your hobby? That you spend so much time taking part in indoor cycling classes you could lead them and get paid. The friend who lays that niggling seed of an idea, which at first you swiftly bat away, but then somehow without truly understanding why you've acted on it.

That was in 2012 when somehow, via a social media channel, Izabela chose to attend my small independent Indoor Cycling Certification Course to learn the art of riding a bike that goes nowhere and creating a class experience. A good instructor needs a few common traits, passion, energy, an open mind, and a willingness to adapt and evolve. I could tell immediately that Izabela had these traits and was on a mission. If a jobs worth doing it's worth doing right.

However some people don't see being an indoor cycling instructor as a real job. Anyone can sit on a bike that goes nowhere and play some music, I've heard it numerous times in my history. Yet within the pages of this book you will discover it isn't actually as easy as all that, and luckily Izabela has noted them down. She has captured unique moments in her teaching career which will resonate with all instructors on the whole. 'Oh it's not just me then,' to the 'Why haven't I thought of that?'

We get up on the lead bike and have the ability to impact people's lives every day. With the aid of this book my fellow instructors, you can ensure it is more likely to be a positive impact.

Neil Troutman
Velocity Indoor Cycling Program

Dedication

For Karolina, the best sister one could wish for.

Acknowledgement

"I want to thank EVERYONE who ever said anything positive to me or taught me something. I heard it all, and it meant something".

Tiffany Haddish the American actress, comedian and author wrote these words in her autobiography. This really resonated with me and I would like to thank anybody who has ever helped me find a new class to teach, or gave me a chance to cover for them, as this is how I got 95% of my classes over the years. This is how I honed my craft and was able to write this book.

I would also like to thank all the studios where I failed my auditions over the years. This only made me more determined as an instructor to prove my worth.

Thank you to my fellow instructors I have become friends with over the years.

Inka Goodwin – it's your fault I even decided to qualify as an instructor.

Cheryl Browne – you introduced me to the Facebook page in 2012 where I got my first class covers from and which I have been using since.

That is where I found Neil Troutman and took his amazing course that really showed me how to teach a cycling class. He became my first mentor and our paths have been intertwined ever since. Thank you for your help with that book, boss (and your suggestion of having illustrations done)!

Obi Ohuruogu – for our inspirational chats over the years about anything fitness.

Serena Sheree – for always keeping it real and funny.

To my riders who have become friends, too and who never let me drop my standards: Morgan, Hannah, Holly, Rachel, Jordan, Nicola, Michelle, Emma, Charlie, Tom, the Coppins and dozens more. For being there for me when I was ill – Bernie, Tony, Briget, Russ and countless others. And to Josh Turner who helped me so much with my Parkinson's project.

To all my professional mentors whose knowledge and expertise have been crucial in getting me where I am: Caesar Russell, Janine Joseph, Doyle Armstrong, James Lamb, Karyn Silenzi. Jennifer Sage and ICA.

Next, we are getting to the core people that were there from the start of the writing process. We spent a few hours laughing at various title ideas (like: "Don't touch my knob – a guide to indoor cycling"), namely Amanda-Jane Kershen and Stevie Barr. You both read many chapters as I was working on them and helped me make the book what it turned out to be. Thank you for your ideas, suggestions and the no nonsense critique.

Now onto the people who fed me throughout the process: The Deli Boutique on St John's Hill. I spent between three and six hours a week for around four months typing furiously at my favourite table while Andrea and William brought me countless croissants with jam, coffees, and full English, all prepared with a smile by Eros – grazie. Thank you for not chucking me out!

Thank you to my publisher Choir Press who I found through a Google search, but who turned out to be the perfect choice. Miles and the whole team – you have helped my dream come true.

Thank you to my illustrator Simon Goodway.

Finally, onto the most important person in my life who always keeps me grounded and drives me mad by making sing-a-song about everything (oh, yes, she can). My youngest sister who has taken care of me through my cancer treatment despite having her own health issues. For making me laugh at the worst of times. And for her feedback on this book (your sentences are too long). Love you Baba!

Contents

Introduction		ix
About Me		xiii
Chapter 1	Confessions of a Cover Girl or Words of Wisdom for New Instructors	1
Chapter 2	Fiascos	11
Chapter 3	Keeping Track	19
Chapter 4	Health and Safety Concerns	25
Chapter 5	Instructors' Dilemmas	37
Chapter 6	Class Profiles	50
Chapter 7	Music	56
Chapter 8	How to Put Bums on Seats and Keep Your Classes Busy	62
Chapter 9	Teaching Styles	73
Chapter 10	Feedback Forms	80
Chapter 11	Keeping It Real	82
Chapter 12	Intensity	95
Chapter 13	Using Notes	104
Chapter 14	Motivating the Riders	108
Chapter 15	Special Populations	115
Chapter 16	Auditions	122
Chapter 17	Studio Logistics	134
Chapter 18	Gym Wear	139
Chapter 19	Hygiene in the Studio	143
Chapter 20	Say WHAT?!	146

Ride and Shine – How to become a Successful Cycling (or Group Exercise) Instructor.

All the questions you need answers to after *your certification course.*

Introduction

Why did I write this book?

Despite years of experience, there are still many things I come across in my journey as an indoor cycling instructor that stop me in my tracks. Some are learning 'lightbulb moments' that expand my teaching toolbox, others are things so surprising that I need to pick my jaw up off the floor before I can move on. I know that if these moments happen to me, they must be happening to others so why not share them?

Over the years, especially when I started teaching, I have searched for a book that would cover all the basics but could find nothing. The closest I got is the amazing Indoor Cycling Association's website which I use regularly.

This book may prepare less experienced instructors for what they may face, make them think twice or simply make them laugh.

To share my teaching experiences, both successes and fiascos, with other instructors I joined a few social media pages, groups and forums. They are a real gold mine of group exercise instructor know-how. You can learn a lot from others and develop professional, even mentoring, relationships that will stay with you forever regardless of where in the world they are based.

A couple of years ago I was almost addicted to trawling the endless posts on social media, getting frustrated when the same questions were being asked multiple times. Were people not paying attention? Why ask the same thing over and over?

That is when I thought: if only there was a place where those most popular questions and answers were available at any time, without having to scroll down through hundreds of posts on various pages.

This was the moment the idea for this book was born, but I was sitting on it for a good couple of years always distracted by life.

Then in 2018 I was diagnosed with breast cancer and that made me reassess my life and my priorities. Faced with a very uncertain future I looked at myself in the mirror and said: 'you have been thinking about writing this book for so long. What are you waiting for?' From then on, every Tuesday and Friday I would go to my local café and spend two to three hours writing (fuelled by fresh French croissants and the best coffee in London).

You are now holding in your hands the final product that I am very proud of. And if you find a few pastry crumbs between the pages, you will know how they got there.

Who is this book for?

This book is relevant particularly to indoor cycling instructors; however, any group exercise instructor will find something they can learn or relate to in here.

It will also make a great read for someone who regularly participates in group exercise classes giving them a unique insight into what it is like to be on the other side of the studio.

What will you find here?

You will find many most frequently asked questions and descriptions of various situations you may encounter in your teaching experience as a new (or seasoned) indoor cycling or group exercise instructor. Because, let's be honest, however great your initial qualification, however long the training course, dozens of questions will only arise when you leave the classroom and face a group of random people that you are now responsible for. At this point, you may feel alone and think: 'I bet this has only happened to me!' Rest assured that, as one instructor put it, it is not the case:

So, it isn't just me. Others seem to have the same problem. I thought maybe it's the same students that travel around the country to torture cycle instructors.

Where do the answers come from?

Mainly from my own experience, conversations with my colleagues and from social media forums. I have been collating them for years.

Some for their content value others purely because they are hilarious.

Disclaimer: I have not set out to belittle anyone or bash any teaching style in indoor cycling. You may not agree with some of the things you find in here, and that is fine. In the end, we as instructors are on a never-ending journey of development. My teaching style today is a world away from what it was at the start. If your experience is different from mine, I have no problem with it, and neither should you.

Will I find definitive answers to all the questions asked here?

In many cases there is no right or wrong (or definitive) answer. There are many ways to skin a cat. Unless we talk about science, that is.

Some of the questions may have more than one answer. Some answers will start from, 'it depends'. Some controversial ones may have opposing answers included just to make you think and choose the one that agrees with who you are as a person and as an instructor.

How to read this book?

You can go cover to cover or look at the contents table and head straight to the section that interests you.

All that's left now is to clip in, put some comfortable resistance on and enjoy the ride!

About Me

I was not particularly sporty as a child, but I had a bike – everyone did then. During my university years in the mid to late 90s there were no gyms or gym culture in Poland, but every summer I would go to work in Italy for around two months cleaning and washing dishes in hotels. Then my partner in crime Joanna and I would go out dancing all night every night.

When I moved to the UK in 2000, I discovered salsa dancing and quickly became addicted, taking eight classes a week and dancing at every opportunity. That surely kept me fit.

Then in about 2008 I got this idea to run a marathon, so my friend Magda and I started training and a year later completed the Edinburgh marathon. I really got the running, or rather jogging bug, but my back had a different view on it and in the end, I had surgery which put a stop to my running.

At that point, I was qualified as a Level three personal trainer and would take cycling classes as a participant. My friend Inka who was an indoor cycling instructor at my gym told me I should become an instructor. She said: 'You are taking the classes regularly anyway; you may as well get paid for teaching them'. And that is how I stumbled upon my dream job that would combine my love of cycling and my real-life passion – teaching. Thank you, Inka.

Teaching was on the cards all along. In the late 90s I spent a couple of years working as a primary school teacher. I loved teaching kids new skills, but struggled with all the other things that the process of working with seven to 14-year-olds entailed. When I found indoor cycling, I could combine my love for cycling with a passion for educating without the stress of practically parenting someone for a few hours a day.

I have been teaching indoor cycling since 2012 and at the time of writing this book I have taught over 2,500 classes. I have taught at small private gyms, big chain and corporate gyms, and boutique studios. I have worked on bikes with no data, some data, power meters, and consoles as well as PIQ and big integrated screens streaming videos and data in real time. You name an indoor bike, and I have probably taught on it.

Over the years I have completed various courses, certifications, took part in webinars, workshops and attended live conferences on indoor cycling and fitness yet I find there is still so much for me to learn.

Sadly, being an instructor doesn't pay well enough, so I also work part-time as an accountant and occasionally as a sports massage therapist, but I live and breathe indoor cycling.

I don't cycle outdoors regularly but I have travelled across a few countries on cycling holidays: Spain, Holland, Costa Rica, Colombia and Peru, so I have experienced steep gradients, fast descents and cycling at high altitude. I took part in a few sportives, but purely for the challenge of completing them (Etape Loch Ness, Tour of Cambridge, London to Brighton). All these experiences have been key in my becoming a better instructor.

CHAPTER 1:
Confessions of a Cover Girl or Words of Wisdom for New Instructors

Preparation Part 1 (things you can control)

Being a new instructor or one that takes on numerous cover classes in various places, can be very daunting. You don't know the crowd. You are still mastering your craft and it can get very stressful, especially when things go wrong so eliminating as many risks as possible is the key to your preparation. Many things can go wrong, so you want to make sure you tick off as many points off your checklist as possible.

I am a big believer in checklists – either mental or those you can have on your phone or in your diary. Until heading off to teach becomes your second nature, it can be very helpful to use some form of a checklist. This chapter will introduce you to two of these.

Before we discuss profile or playlist choice, let's focus on the inanimate objects that can make or break your class.

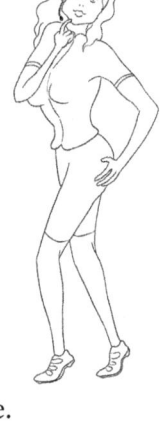

Checklist #1: Instructor's bag of wonders

Whether you choose to have a special bag, a box or have a section in your usual gym bag for these items, you should never head to teach a class without the following:

- ✓ Aux cable and new iPhone/iPod extension
- ✓ Various size microphone windshields
- ✓ Batteries: AA, AAA, 9V
- ✓ Microphone belt or a cycling top with a pocket
- ✓ Back up device with an emergency playlist
- ✓ Basic Allen key (to free stuck cleats)

- ✓ Hair band (great to hold an oversized mic shield in place)
- ✓ Small towel (some gyms may not provide them)
- ✓ Optional: marker that can be used on mirrors/windows (to write class plan)

I think there is no need for further explanation of what these items are so let's just focus on why having those items with you at all times, gives you a peace of mind.

Aux cable missing or not compatible

These days many studios use Bluetooth technology and most gyms have got the aux leads attached to the system, but bear in mind that Bluetooth connection may be temperamental. Sometimes the cable provided by the gym is a bit of a loose fit which will influence the sound quality.

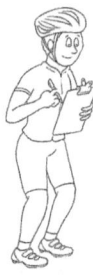

TACKLE STRATEGY: Have your own aux cable. Or check in advance if you can use Bluetooth technology to connect your device. And if you play music from your phone, what with Apple making sure every new phone becomes incompatible with your old headphones etc, make sure that before you change over to the new one, you have purchased the right attachment so you can still connect to the sound system. Even if the system uses Bluetooth, things can go wrong so have that cable always in your bag.

Mic belts and windshields

You turn up to a studio and these items are not available. You have no pocket for the mic and there is no way of attaching the box to your clothing.

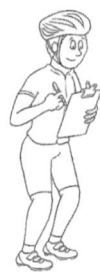

TACKLE STRATEGY: please, have your own. We are all (mostly) self-employed and these are business expenses. Wash the belt and the windshields regularly. I have two belts I alternate and a whole heap of windshields. One lasts me a few months, but I wash it after or before every class using soap, hot water and dry I it under the hand dryer. Check your bag every day. These are not to be forgotten.

Do not underestimate the importance of these little suckers. If you don't understand why you need them, take a class as a participant with an instructor who shies away from using them. You're welcome.

Vile alert! There are gyms that try to help instructors by providing these items. You go to the cupboard, open the CYCLE STUDIO box and there is the belt and the little sponge on the mouthpiece.

When I see these through the box lid, I brace myself and stand a safe distance away from it holding my breath as I open the box to retrieve them, *leaving* the sponge and the belt behind and closing the lid *before* I breathe in again.

Why would you use these, drench them in sweat and saliva and lock them still wet in a box?! They become chemical waste! I would rather hold the mic in my hand then use a belt that smells like a dead animal.

Microphone batteries missing

Yeah, we have all been there. It's 50/50 these days with gyms providing batteries or having the rechargeable ones, and the ones with microphones with empty spaces where the suckers should be. Or your worst nightmare – the mics with the weird 9V battery that is so uncommon you have not used it before.

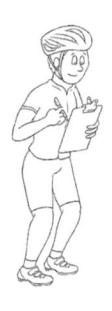

TACKLE STRATEGY: always carry two or four AA batteries and one of the 9V ones. And a bit of science here, as I swear to God some instructors don't realise it: if a microphone (or any battery-operated equipment) takes two batteries and upon switching the ON button the thing has flat-lined, you cannot just replace one! You need to change both. Do you remember the science class when they explained this?!

Even if the battery is rechargeable but the previous user did not connect it to the charger, coming 15 minutes early and connecting it then may be the difference between having to yell for 45 minutes or not.

Note: batteries can go dead if you keep them in your bag next to items like a mobile phone so check them from time to time.

Towelgate

I sweat profusely. I swear sometimes it feels like a Pavlov's dog response: I hear music and my body starts sweating in preparation. I categorically must have a towel over my handlebars and in most gyms across London, it is provided as standard, but it is worth asking about when you agree to cover somewhere new or carry your own just in case. Especially since many studios no longer have dry paper towels leaving you no alternative (and nicking a whole roll of toilet paper may be frowned upon). Oh, and even if there is a shop next door where you can buy a towel; trust me, I have done that too and can confirm that a new towel, before it's washed for the first time, does *not* absorb any sweat ...

Preparation Part 2 – Profile and Music Choice

How do you choose your class profile and playlist for a cover class? (or your first class in a new studio)

It goes without saying that you should have your **profile** and **music** planned for every session, preferably including a contingency plan (especially for a one-off cover class).

It is important to resist the temptation to think: '*I will teach the hardest class ever. I will show them what a badass instructor I am!*' and approach the situation more methodically to ensure the best possible experience for both sides.

First, when taking on a cover, ask the regular instructor what they normally do in their sessions. Do people ask me? Not often. Do I ask? Always.

Checklist #2: What do I ask about?

- ✓ What bikes are there (data or none)?
- ✓ What format do you usually teach? (HIT, endurance, etc.)
- ✓ Do you ever play long tracks (like 7–10 minutes)?
- ✓ What kind of music do you play?

I make my choice of profile based on the answers, yet I always have plan B.

First, if you take on a new class or have no contact with the regular instructor, something current in terms of music or a varied playlist are the way to go. Avoid going heavy on one artist or one genre or it may all backfire.

Second, the profile should be adaptable to whatever the demographics of the group in front of you. Short to medium length intervals are always a safe choice. Even if your regulars love riding long intervals (around 10 minutes) it does not mean every group will appreciate them.

Fail to plan, plan to fail – know your environment

And now onto the other things that every instructor heading to a new venue should consider. Set yourself up for success by anticipating potential hazards.

If you only teach at your regular places, you know your ins and outs. You know what can possibly go wrong and who to ask for help. But if you are adventurous and prepared to cover at various locations, or if you are new to the venue, the possibilities of what may go wrong are numerous. Here are some examples of disaster scenarios you should be prepared for as they have all happened to me.

Is this the right place?

If you have just thought: 'Really? You surely know where you agreed to teach!' trust me, it can go wrong. It happened to me a couple of times that I thought I knew which site we were talking about only to realise that was not the case when I arrived at the gym. There were a few sites of the same chain close by and I got them wrong. Thankfully the right one was just around the corner.

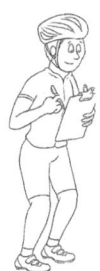

TACKLE STRATEGY: if you are heading towards a new area, make sure you check the map beforehand and allow extra time just in case. Do you know how to get there if the route you planned fails? What if the tube (subway in the US) is not working? Any delay due to transport will cause you additional stress. At least if you have everything else organised you are still winning.

No gym management or riders will look at you favourably if you rock up 15 minutes late.

Sound system you have never seen before

This one applies mainly to new instructors. It used to be my greatest fear – what if I don't know what to press, or if there is a secret button somewhere in the back room (most often with *'power'* written on it)?

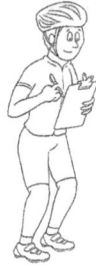

TACKLE STRATEGY: get there early. And I mean like 30 minutes early if this is your first visit. If a class is taking place when you arrive, make sure you ask the instructor before they leave, if there are any tricks you need to know. If the room is empty and things do not work, you may need to find a manager or a studio coordinator or The One Who Knows the Sound System. If the venue is big, it may take time so allow for it.

Beware of Wi-Fi wreaking havoc with your playlist!

I know some people stream their music using Wi-Fi. I used to do that myself. Then once, in the middle of the class, I realised the song that had started was supposed to be coming on much later. What the … – I looked at the iPad and saw that five songs went *online* and would need to play from iCloud which for some reason wasn't picking up. I could only play three out of ten songs from that playlist!

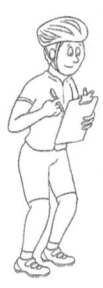

TACKLE STRATEGY: Download your playlists onto your device so you are not dependant on Wi-Fi connectivity.

Alternatively, have an extra couple of playlists at the ready. My profile that day was supposed to be a 15-minute climb. We did the first song, but I needed 10 more minutes. I simply went to the next playlist with 'hill' in the title and used those songs. That is why putting music into categories or naming your playlists appropriately is crucial (see chapter on Music).

If possible, have a back-up device. Once during a 60-minute ride that I didn't use for a few weeks I realised that one important song had disappeared but I knew I had it on my phone so I made a joke to the group saying that they were about to witness my smooth sound engineering skills where I would be changing music devices half way through the ride but it worked!

You turn up to find bikes (or PIQ system) you have never seen before

If the information on bike and visual systems is not offered when you take on a class, then ask. You don't want to look unprofessional in front of the riders. If you cannot obtain the information in advance, you will need to make a decision whether to use it once you get into the studio.

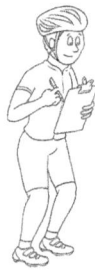

TACKLE STRATEGY: turning up early comes handy again. Sometimes locating the right levers to change the bike set up may be a challenge, let alone operating PIQ systems. When it comes to visual systems like My Ride or Spivi, you can always tell the riders that you are just covering and will keep them busy without using visuals.

If it is just a system showing RPM, Watts, etc., and you know how to switch it on, do so if required. But never feel pressured: if you don't know what visuals the system will play, do not switch them on as they may not match your class at all and cause confusion.

This is all wrong!

Imagine that you asked all the right questions and were told the bikes have power meters, the group is really into serious training, there are many cyclists etc., so you decided to do a profile using power zones.

On the day you walk into the studio and yes, the consoles show RPM but not the power (or they are not calibrated so the numbers are all over the place). As the riders start filing in you get one outdoor lycra-clad cyclist, three people who have clearly never been on a bike before, four who have no idea about the set-up and when you say 'RPM' they look at you as if you were an alien, so you abort the mission of teaching with power.

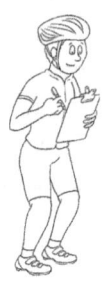

TACKLE STRATEGY: PLAN B! Always have it. It doesn't have to be an easier class intensity-wise, but your teaching and cueing approach will be totally different. You can challenge yourself and still use the profile you planned but use RPE (Rate of Perceived Exertion) as the only teaching tool.

Even if you have a regular class relying heavily on technology, would you be able to teach 'old school' if the technology failed? I teach in a 40-bike studio full of IC6 bikes with consoles but for a few weeks there was a serious technical glitch and 50 percent of the consoles would go dead after a few minutes of riding. I was glad that I had started teaching all those years ago on 'bare bikes' with no data feedback as I could revert to that experience.

Cycling shoes

As instructors, I assume 99% of us wear cycling shoes when teaching; however, even though 99% of bikes have the standard MTB cleats, some boutique studios have the road shoe cleats. Sometimes you can turn the pedal over for MTB cleat but there may be times when you cannot use your own shoes. These places usually have their own shoes you can rent.

To me it is a nightmare as wearing someone else's shoes – no matter how well disinfected – is my worst-case scenario. Plus, if you are not used to the road shoe cleats, good luck walking around the studio. Just saying …

There is nothing you can do in that case. Embrace the experience and think happy thoughts.

Preparation Part 3 – Because Life Happens

And who are you?!

When I used to be a gym member, I had my favourite instructors just like everyone else. I was looking forward to their classes knowing what to expect.

Then every so often I would turn up, set up my bike and another instructor would walk in. If I had never seen them before I would get very anxious thinking 'Oh no, here we go! What will their class be like? Should I stay or should I go?'. I must admit a few times I would just see the 'wrong' instructor walk in and I would walk out …

Karma is a b**** though and a few years later I found myself on the receiving end of the said treatment. If you are a newly qualified instructor, you cannot help but take this kind of behaviour personally. The two worst-case scenarios are: when people sit through the first 10 minutes of your class and then leave because they had a chance to see what you are all about and decided it was not worth their time or when they heckle you loudly, try to undermine you and are being generally obnoxious. Thankfully, the latter has never happened to me.

You cannot help how you feel when this happens, but you do learn with experience that it doesn't mean that your class was awful. It just was so different from the usual, they couldn't deal with it. In my opinion it is better for someone who does not enjoy it to leave, than if they were to sit there, sighing and rolling their eyes or doing their own thing and completely ignoring your instructions.

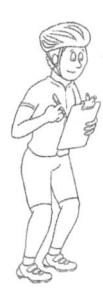

TACKLE STRATEGY: as you walk in, smile and say hello. If you see consternation on people's faces say stuff like: 'No, I am clearly not John, but you will still get a great class'. Walk around offering help and asking what they usually do or if you had done your research then say it. This will show your respect for the group and will change some people's minds about leaving before you even begin.

Talking to people as they file into the studio may also help you make up your mind whether to go with plan A or B.

If I see people battling internally or hovering around the doors, I say: 'Please come in. I know you weren't expecting me, but I can guarantee you will get a great workout. Let's make a deal. If after 10 minutes you think that this is not your thing, please feel free to leave. But you are here now, you planned to attend this session so give it a go.'

How much do you care about the participants in the one-off/cover classes?

This one is tricky. I *always* care about people I teach even if I think I may never see them again. If they have a bad form, I will correct them. I also go through the bike set up in every single class.

However, the following situation happened a few years back which was a major learning curve. I agreed to cover a class for three consecutive weeks. Those riders had no clue about bike set up and their postures were clearly never corrected. I was horrified and so with good intentions, I ended up practically criticising them for 45 minutes.

I realised at the end of the class that nobody was smiling, and I was mentally exhausted. A week later when I came into the studio, one woman who was already set up greeted me with: 'Oh no!' and left. That was a tough lesson in letting go: you cannot correct a lifetime of bad habits in one class and if you keep correcting all the time, you will put people off.

Pick your battles.

Is it normal to lose sleep over classes?

To quote the great Homer Simpson: 'DUH!'

Before I taught my first ever class, I was waking up every hour on the hour worrying I would oversleep. I got up exhausted, but the adrenaline kicked in as soon as I got into that studio.

Now every time I start a new permanent class or even every time I am supposed to cover a class somewhere I have never taught before, I get the jitters. I don't lose sleep over it that much – unless it's an early morning class as I always panic that I will not wake up in time, so I wake up multiple times during the night.

Despite over 2,500 classes taught, when I walk into a studio to face a group of complete strangers, I have butterflies in my stomach and get a real adrenaline rush. I think it must be what a performer who is about to go on stage in front of live audience feels. You want to do well but you don't know what the audience's reaction is going to be. What if they don't like it?

I think slight jitters are a good thing. It means that regardless of how many years you have been doing it for, you still care and want to make sure that every class you deliver is as good as it can be.

CHAPTER 2

Fiascos

This chapter links to the previous one about preparation but all scenarios described here are about facing situations that are beyond your control, all bar one.

The sound system not working

There is no music, or you need to use the old boombox in the corner or worse still, I have just seen an instructor sharing on a forum that their colleague locked the cupboard with the stereo and took the key with them by mistake so there was no way to use the sound system.

That's a tough one. I had the Boombox (usually the Aqua class stereo) experience a few times but have never done a silent class. However, on the bikes with monitors, I see no major problem. The only thing in this scenario is that your cueing and the use of RPE (rate of perceived exertion) must be on point.

Have you ever thought about what you would do in such a situation? If your classes are driven by music – you go with the chorus and verse flow rather than have a structured plan – this may be a mission impossible.

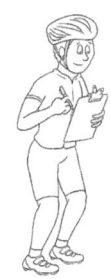

TACKLE STRATEGY: I don't think anyone can make you start a class if the music does not work. It may be down to you to decide.
If the sound system is faulty, for example there is no bass, and your class plan relies heavily on music, it may spoil the whole feel and flow of the class. Do your best in the circumstances.

I had to teach five classes a week at a place where there was no bass (just a horrible thumping sound) for eight consecutive weeks. My choice was to either not use any music or choose songs that did not have much bass in them. I went with option two, but trust me, it was not an easy task as that's a pretty limited number of songs in my library.

If the sound system does not work, some gyms will cancel a cycling class. However, if the issue occurs shortly before the class, it may not always be possible to contact the members so they may leave the decision to you: can you teach without music?

In this case, the decision will be yours and yours alone. It will depend on your teaching style, experience and may be heavily influenced by the bikes you teach on.

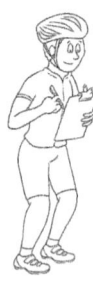

TACKLE STRATEGY: Be prepared that even if you decide to bite the bullet, some people may leave the room when they realise there will be no music.

If you have bikes with consoles showing RPM and power and have a power target-based profile up your sleeve where music just enhances the experience but is not the main driver, you simply conduct the class purely by the numbers and RPE.

Such a class would however expose you as a coach: can you motivate and lead a class just with your voice? You could even allow people to use their own music and headphones (if they still follow your instructions). You just need to use visual cues to mark the start and end of an interval.

If the bikes have no consoles, the task will get much more complicated and I would not be surprised if nobody wanted to stay.

To sum up, always have a few extra playlists on your device so you have options and can choose the lesser evil. I would also recommend always having one profile that is based purely on timed intervals and intensity (or you can improvise one). And be prepared for sounds of loud breathing.

Mic not working or no mic at all

A variation of the above problem would be a perfectly working sound system but no microphone.

Many instructors, mainly new ones, are known to say: 'I don't need/use a mic. I just use my voice. I am loud as it is.'

First, let me say that I used to be the same. At the start of your career you think you are invincible. But a couple of thousands of classes later I have changed my tune – pun intended. After years of teaching, being loud and getting excited cueing every sprint, my voice has suffered considerably. I can no longer even do karaoke or belt out my favourite songs when in the shower because my voice cracks straight away.

These days I refuse to teach in studios without a mic and have been known to bring sheets of paper with SHOULDERS DOWN, RELAX YOUR GRIP etc printed on them to hold up, when my voice is poorly.

There are workshops teaching breathing techniques and voice projection which are always good to explore. I would also recommend you checking out Fitness Career Mastery podcasts, especially episodes 45, 46, and 79 on voice physiology and psychology to fully appreciate the power of this most important tool of any group exercise instructor.

If you are still convinced that you do *not* need a mic, please take a class with an instructor who doesn't use it, either. Preferably in a big studio with 30–40 bikes and make sure you sit at the back. You will gain an appreciation for a mic no third-party advice could convince you of.

Using a mic will allow you to develop and enhance your teaching skills like coaching using calm and steady voice, visualisations, stories, open questions, etc., instead of only yelling short commands.

Without a working mic, you may need to change your plan as far as the profile is concerned. If you planned an endurance ride with visualisations, focused on eliciting intrinsic motivation which would require you to talk with a calm tone of voice, it would not work without a microphone. Particularly in a big studio. Certain cues are not meant to be shouted.

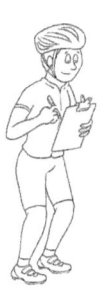

TACKLE STRATEGIES: I have an ace up my sleeve for situations like that. As a Stages Cycling UK ambassador, I was given a lovely cowbell with my name engraved on it. I swear to you that after my iPad and microphone shields this is the most important item that is in my bag. I have gained fame as The One with the Bell. I use it in almost every class to mark the start and end of the interval, to mark the final minute of an interval, I ring it for the final 10 seconds of a long interval, you name it. It saves my voice and brings a great vibe to the class. It's particularly handy when mic troubles occur. You can get your own bell or even one of those fog horns associated with cycling competitions. I used to have one, but I prefer the bell.

To save my voice and any confusion, before I turn on the music, I explain how I will be using the bell so everyone can hear me. Even if you don't have a bell, explain the structure of the class clearly before you press play. And when necessary, lower the volume in the recovery tracks to explain the upcoming section or interval.

I know that whenever I need to yell in a class, if the microphone is not working, I get exhausted very quickly and if I do high intensity efforts with my riders, just shouting: 3,2,1! to mark the end of one, makes me feel lightheaded.

Remember to be kind to your voice and minimise the damage to it. You cannot foresee technical issues but always ask if the gym has a working microphone and what batteries you need.

Air con not working

When the air conditioning is not working or is not strong enough for the size of the studio and the number of riders, it is imperative to take steps to ensure the riders' safety.

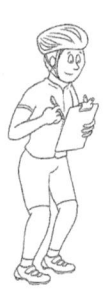

TACKLE STRATEGIES: Whenever possible try and get the gym to arrange a fan or two. See if there is an option of opening a window and/or keeping the door to the studio open – which may not always be the case due to noise levels.

Failing all that, explain as people are filing in that they need water and if they forgot their bottle they should go and purchase one before the start.

It is imperative to explain to the riders that should they feel that they are overheating or getting dizzy, they should take a break, and should they struggle too much with the heat, they are free to leave early.

Ensure you make this clear to any pregnant women in your class!

In such situations I often change the plan in favour of lower intensity longer intervals at moderate effort and I have been known to even postpone a long-planned FTP test session due to the excessive temperature in the studio.

I advise riders that they should drink as much as they need and should they run out of water, they can wave their bottle and I will go and refill it for them. I do that even if the closest tap is outside of the studio. This is what I am comfortable with and many riders take me up on that offer grateful that they don't have to break their rhythm. Others choose to leave the studio and have a cooling break as they refill their bottles.

OMFG! I was supposed to teach today?! When you didn't turn up to the class you agreed to cover

We are only humans hence we are not perfect, which means that sooner or later a mistake is bound to happen. And the risk factor grows exponentially to the number of classes you take on, especially the one-offs. However, I am inclined to say that the higher the number of years of experience, the more reliable the instructor.

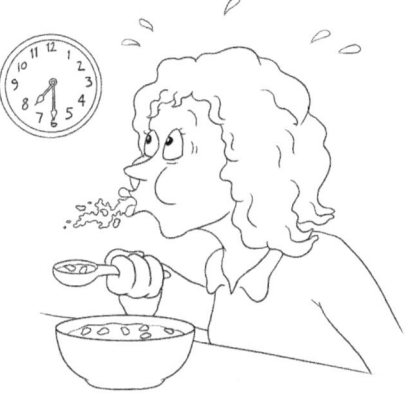

First time I failed (and it has happened twice in my seven-year career) was when my close friend asked me to cover a 6:45am class at my local gym located about 10 minutes' walk from my house. The class was around Easter time, but she had asked me a couple of months in advance. I put it down in my calendar on the kitchen wall.

On the day in question, I woke up around 5:30am (with no alarm set) but couldn't work out why so I went back to sleep. I got up at 7am and as I was having breakfast it suddenly hit me: 'I was supposed to teach today!!!'

I cannot quote the exact words I uttered at the realisation. I immediately called the gym to apologise and vent (slightly) that nobody called me, even at 6:45am, as it would have taken me 15 minutes to get dressed and reach the gym so the riders would still get a 30-minute class instead of leaving angry and disappointed.

Thankfully I had been teaching at that gym for over a year by then and they knew I was reliable, and this was just a freak incident. Still, I felt so bad that I would start all classes I taught there that week by apologising to anyone who was left angry that morning.

The second time was again a one-off around Easter or Christmas when *again* I had agreed to cover a class many weeks in advance, then did not set up a proper reminder for myself.

The consequences of you missing the class may be dire. If the gym has no in-house staff to take over and teach the group, the riders may have no other option but go home and I guarantee they will let the reception staff know exactly how they feel about it especially if it's an early morning slot or if there is no other class at the time that they could switch to.

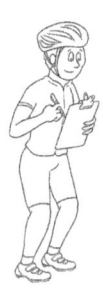

TACKLE STRATEGIES:
Minimise the risk
Firstly, I have learnt my lesson and I avoid agreeing to cover a class too far in advance. Things change, you cannot guarantee you will not be injured or travelling etc. 3–4 weeks is the maximum for me. The main issue is that if you agree to cover a series of classes let's say three months in advance and in the meantime get a permanent class at the same time slot, it is now down to you to find a replacement which can be a lot of hassle. Similarly, I never look for a cover of my classes too early.

Secondly, I mark anything that I agree to cover or take on in my Outlook calendar with reminders a day before, on top of entering the class on my weekly and monthly schedule that I keep (see chapter on Keeping Track). Any classes out of the ordinary are marked in bright colours.

Thirdly, if you asked someone to cover for you, especially if you don't know them well, make sure you message them or call them the day before with a reminder. One of my colleagues who I cover for a few times a year has a habit that always makes me smile. The day before the class he always sends me a message: 'Enjoy the class tomorrow!' Or, 'Work them hard tomorrow', which a nice and indirect way of saying, 'Don't forget to haul you're a*** to my class tomorrow'.

If you are going to be away for a week or more or travelling in a different time zone, just send a reminder of the full schedule to the respective instructors a few days earlier. Better safe than sorry.

If it does happen

If you oversleep or are running late, do your best to contact the gym or any of your regular riders if you have their details. It helps if you are known for your reliability, as people will wait for you if you had enough respect to let them know you are on your way.

Once, after two weeks holiday, I turned up at the gym for 6:45am class. In fact, I got there so early due to jet lag, that the gym was still closed, and I managed to get in with the cleaners. I set up the bike and the music but at 6:30am as people started to come in, I remember thinking it was odd to have so many new faces. Then a woman walked into the studio very purposefully, approached me and the following dialogue ensued:

Woman: 'Excuse me, and who are you?'
Me (realising she was an instructor): 'Sorry, what day is it today? It is Tuesday, right?'
Woman: 'No, it's Thursday and this is my class.'
Me: '$*$! *!'

I *was* teaching that day. And at 6:45am. At a different gym! I have never packed my stuff so fast in my life. Running down the steps in my cycling shoes (thank God these were MTB cleats and not roadies) I ran up the road to a bus stop. Thankfully the other gym was only four stops away and I called them from the bus asking the receptionist to tell the riders I was on my way. I ran into the studio sweaty and out of breath to find 30 or so riders calmly warming up. They have never seen me late so were more than happy to forgive me.

Own up

> 'I feel like such a jerk – I signed up to sub for a class this morning, and completely forgot! Any thoughts on how to make up for it? Or is it best to simply apologise, thank the person for covering for me, and just move on?"

It is more stressful if you don't turn up to cover somebody else's class as the world of fitness is small and you don't want to gain fame as the unreliable one. If possible, be the first one to contact the instructor you promised to cover and the gym directly, not to get blacklisted.

If you cannot make the early morning class – emergencies

I went on a weekend away once and was due to fly back on Monday evening. My first class was on Tuesday morning at 6:30am and it was always a busy one with over 20 riders. Unfortunately, my first flight was delayed making me lose my connection and consequently I was put on the 7:30am flight the following morning.

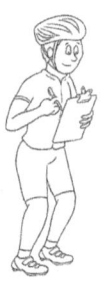

TACKLE STRATEGY: Life happens but to minimise the possible risk I should have got that class covered before I went away. But I did not, so I had to minimise the damage.

I knew about 7pm on Monday there was a risk of me not making it to the Tuesday morning class, so I used our WhatsApp group to try and get cover but had no luck. I wanted to inform the reception staff so they could tell members as they were arriving in the morning the class was cancelled and to prepare them for a possible backlash but there was no way of me doing it.

And here the good old social media came in handy. Many of my regulars follow me on there so I sent messages to as many as I could. I also posted in my status that the class was not on. But the friendship I have developed with our cleaner was what helped me the most. Knowing that he would be at the gym even before the reception staff, I texted him asking to pass the message on.

It's about who you know in life!

CHAPTER 3
Keeping Track

I wasn't born holding an abacus. I always joke that if A-levels in maths were compulsory, I would still be in secondary school, but after over 10 years of working as an accountant I learnt the importance of cash flow and credit control which is basically keeping tabs on where your money is, how much you are owed, where the payments are coming from and when.

Ninety-nine percent of gyms and studios in the UK want their instructors to be self-employed freelancers. That means that you get paid a gross amount and it is your duty to pay the tax on it by submitting a tax return by the end of the tax year. I am not familiar with other countries' taxation systems so I can only talk about the UK.

In a nutshell

In the UK the tax year runs from 5 April until 6 April. You need to submit your tax return by 31 October (if filing paper version) and by 31 January if you do it online. Any tax must be paid by 31 January.

If your tax liability for the year is more than £1,000, you will also need to make two payments on account for the new tax year. 50% by 31 January and 50% by 31 July. I don't want to go into more details here, HMRC website offers all necessary information. Simply search for self-assessment.

Can I do it myself?

People get scared when it comes to filing their tax return and I often get asked: Do I need an accountant? It depends on a few things:

- Are your tax affairs straightforward? Are you only a self-employed sole trader for the purposes of teaching classes with maybe another full-time or part-time job? If this is the case, you should be able to handle your taxes yourself.

- Are you a limited company director or do you get income from properties or shares? I would go with an accountant unless you really know what you are doing.
- Do you lease premises or equipment, or subcontract your work? Get advice from an accountant.
- Do you struggle keeping track of your bills and receipts? Do you keep meticulous record of your income? If this side of the business is your weakness, then get an accountant.

If you are just a one-man-band and you are systematic in keeping records of monies in and monies out, then you should be fine filing your tax return on your own. HMRC has many free of charge interactive webinars available all year round where you can learn about expenses, tax free allowances etc. Just sign up for this service and you will start getting e-mails with dates and times. These are much better than trying to call the helpline which often means over 30 minutes of being on hold.

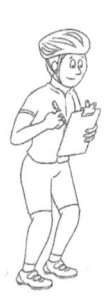

TACKLING STRATEGY: If you decide to handle the tax affairs yourself, meticulous record keeping is a must.

I keep an Excel spreadsheet that is simple but acts in capacity of a diary of all my classes, their locations, duration, times, fees, payments received, methods of payments, profiles used and business expenses. At any point in time I know my predicted income for the next couple of months, exact income for the current tax year, how much money is due to come into my account, when and from which gym and what tax is due up until now. Mind blowing, right?

This spreadsheet is my bible and it is invaluable when you get paid a wrong amount or to make you realise you did not get paid. Some gyms send a detailed remittance by e-mail before they make the actual payment which makes it easy to reconcile what was due and what was paid. Others just make a payment. Different gyms pay at different times of the month. If you do not keep a tab on what you were due, you may not realise you got underpaid. It is in your own interest to be vigilant.

The spreadsheet I use gives me an instant overview of my earnings and profit in the current tax year and previous years. This is gold when you need to apply for a loan, for example, or if you want to go into a partnership with someone and they want to see a quick snapshot of your finances in the last few years. It shows you how your business has been performing. It also makes it easy to budget in your holidays since when you don't work you don't get paid.

The key to making this spreadsheet perform its function is consistency in updating it. I have been doing it almost daily since the start. All my fixed classes are there. Every time I agree to cover a one-off class, I immediately add it on. If I have a social outing booked it still goes onto the spreadsheet so I know I cannot take on a cover class on that day.

When I get paid, I update the PAID column, so I know if the amount paid was correct. If the amount paid is short, it takes 10 seconds to copy and paste the table into an e-mail and send it off to the gym pointing out the error. No need to go through calendars or do manual calculations.

Every time I have a business expense like buying music, insurance, CPD courses etc., I put it on the expenses tab.

Some of you may say that you are too busy to do that. I would say I am too busy *not* to. I don't want to spend two hours once a month or two days at the end of the year frantically trawling through mountains of receipts hoping I find all the expenses I can deduct.

When you are diligent with this process, you can do your tax return any time you want. I could submit my tax return on 7 April. And with all the calculations done already it only takes five minutes.

I dare you to try it. I see nothing wrong with hiring an accountant, however, you must remember that in the UK if you are a sole trader and only hire an accountant to do your tax return, so for that one-off job, this expense is *not deductible*. If you pay an accountant to do your books all year round, it is a deductible expense.

The spreadsheet is in Excel so the possibilities are endless – add as many columns as you find useful or delete any irrelevant ones. I added the 'profile' one as it helps me plan my quarterly FTP tests. It also means I can be sure I do not run too many FTP sessions in the same week in the same gym. Use of colours is optional – they work for me.

Date	Fee Note	Client	Notes	Total Due	Paid	How	Time	Profiles
Apr–18								
18/04/2018	Wed	FF		20.00	20.00	a/c	19:30	FTP test
19/04/2018	Thu	DL		20.00	20.00	a/c	06:45	Cadence drills
20/04/2018	Fri	FF		20.00	20.00	a/c	06:30	FTP prep 1
21/04/2018	Sat	PRIVATE		200.00	200.00	CASH		
21/04/2018	Sat	QM		10.00	10.00	CASH	18:00	3x9min climbs
22/04/2018	Sun	Putney LC		50.00	50.00	a/c		
26/04/2018	Thu	DL		20.00	20.00	a/c	06:45	
27/04/2018	Fri	FF		20.00	20.00	a/c	06:30	FTP prep 2
27/04/2018	Fri	DL		20.00	20.00	a/c	18:45	
28/04/2018	Sat	Nuffield		20.00	20.00	a/c	13:10	
28/04/2018	Sat	Queen Mother		20.00	20.00	a/c	18:00	
29/04/2018	Sun							
30/04/2018	Mon	PLC EVENT		200.00	200.00	a/c		
				620.00	620.00			
May-18								
01/05/2018	Tue							
02/05/2018	Wed	FF		20.00		a/c	18:30	
03/05/2018	Thu	PLC EVENT		150.00		a/c	18:30	
				170.00	–			
			TOTAL	790.00	620.00	Collected	170.00	TO COLLECT
PAYMENT TERMS:								
Good Vibes	21st of every month							
Virgin	15th of every month							
37 Degrees.	15th of every month							
		Total for FY 16/17		1,500.00				
		Total for FY 17/18		2,500.00		2.87		TAX DUE FOR THIS YEAR
		Total for FY 18/19		790.00				
			TURNOVER	4,790.00				

07/04/2018	Trainline	tickets to ICG audition	35.45
16/04/2018	Karkoa	gym bag	30.00
23/04/2018	Cycology	kit for audition	40.00
26/04/2018	Taxi	ICG audition train station – office	8.00
02/05/2018	Vistaprint	posters for the event	36.86
30/11/2018	Amazon	year-end trophies	34.50
02/12/2018	iTunes	Music	11.75
09/12/2018	Vistaprint	flyers for six weeks programme	19.98
25/01/2019	Amazon	mic shields	7.00
08/02/2019	Travel and subsistence	TP all day audition	25.00
10/02/2019	Spin shoes	Evans cycles	30.00
16/02/2019	iTunes	Music	8.71
26/02/2019	FF CJS	Blackpool fitness conference	25.00
22/02/2019	Blackpool fitness conference	hotel	40.00
22/02/2019	Blackpool fitness conference	return ticket to Blackpool	40.00
	Rent/Internet	home office allowance	**225.00**
	O2	mobile phone (60%)	**158.40**
			775.65
	Rent and Internet:		225
	O2:		158.4

The spreadsheet:

- Column headings are self-explanatory. You can add or delete some as needed.
- Enter value in column PAID when you receive the payment
- Check regularly the difference between the total of the TOTAL DUE and PAID columns. After you get paid by all the gyms these should be equal. If they are not, you got underpaid.
- When you get paid by a gym, if a breakdown was provided then

check it against the spreadsheet. If there was no breakdown, calculate all the fees due for that period and check against the payment. If they agree, you are done. If you get underpaid or overpaid, inform the gym.
- You can see a TOTAL EARNED less TOTAL COLLECTED (paid already) gives you TO COLLECT which are all self-explanatory.
- At the bottom you can see total for previous tax years. I keep a separate tab for every tax year which is my back up for the tax return, but I also keep a master tab that has all my income over the last seven years. Here I can see totals for all the previous years at a glance. It is easy to see what has been happening to your turnover year on year. I also have a TOTAL TURNOVER for all years at the bottom.
- At the bottom I have payment terms for various gyms I work for as they all pay at different times and this way, I know what is coming when.
- There is a TAX DUE field which is my favourite (to know, not to pay). The formula here is TOTAL FOR FY (financial year) less EXPENSES. Expenses total feeds from a separate tab.
- Expenses tab is where I record all deductible expenses: date, supplier, item, amount. The running total at the bottom feeds onto the TAX DUE field on the main tab.

CHAPTER 4

Health and Safety Concerns

I am a child of late 70s and early 80s and the obsession with health and safety everywhere is driving me nuts. Take that story about the nursery that must get the children to wear life vests because they are taking a walk in their local park with a stream nearby …

Still there are genuine safety concerns when it comes to indoor cycling that I understand and call people out on, or simply do not tolerate in my classes and I will ask the riders to leave for not observing the rules. Let's dive straight into specific examples.

Footwear of lack of it

Trainers

Not everyone will wear cycling shoes to class, especially if they are just starting their adventure with indoor cycling. Unless the studio has a policy stating that you must wear cycling shoes or rent them from the studio, you will have most people wear normal trainers. This is not a problem, if you make sure to mention that they **tuck in their shoelaces**. I have witnessed it myself when someone riding in excess of 100 RPM suddenly came to a very abrupt stop when their shoelaces wrapped around the pedal crank. It was horrendous and took absolute ages to untangle. Thankfully the rider sustain no (immediate) injury.

One of my catchphrases is:

> *Please tuck in the shoelaces if you're wearing trainers so you don't go home with a bike attached to your foot.*

Funny trainers

I have no idea what to call these shoes. They were popular a few years back, but I still see them every so often when setting people up. They have very thick soles that are half-moon shaped. They make you sway forwards and backward when you stand and were invented to apparently engage your core better. The main issue is that the soles are so thick they barely fit into the pedal cage and make maintaining proper pedalling technique hard.

When I see those, I always advise people to bring different shoes next time but if they manage to secure the strap on the shoe, they are not the worst-case scenario.

Plimsoles, flip flops, thin sole espadrilles and the barefoot thingies

Plimsoles are the least evil of these three, still they will cause the foot to arch too much when using high resistance and working out of the saddle. I would not however throw anyone out of the studio for wearing these, yet I would advise them to wear sturdier shoes next time if possible.

Flip flops, you ask. Yes, it did happen. You think this would be the worst? Oh boy, are you wrong! The worst-case scenario that has happened to me was the following.

I was teaching my regular class in a 15-bike studio. We have just started the warm-up and despite the dimmed lights I noticed that there was a girl in the second row whose pedal straps seemed to be loose. I continued cueing the group but walked over to her. I switched off the microphone and said: 'Could you please stop pedalling? We need to tighten up the straps on your shoes, so you are safe when you get out of the saddle'. I then crouched to do just that only to realise *she had no shoes on*! Only socks! I was gobsmacked! I looked at her and she looked back sheepishly saying she forgot her trainers but didn't want to miss the class.

It took me a few seconds to get over the initial shock. This was a corporate gym and I really had no idea if I had the right to ask her to leave, which was what I really wanted to do. There was nobody from the management team close by to ask, so I allowed her to stay provided she wouldn't stand up, go easy on the resistance and if her feet were hurting (duh!) she was free to leave at any point. Incredibly, she stayed until the end.

Immediately after the class I asked the management about my right to refuse someone into the studio based on health and safety, and I was told I had a full right to refuse her entry. It was *not* something I would have asked until it happened as it was not something I could imagine in my wildest dreams.

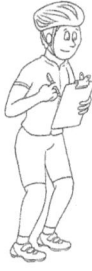

TACKLING STRATEGY: If you know something is a risk, tell the rider. Make sure they understand you told them it was a bad idea. If it is something drastic, like total lack of footwear, you have the right to ask them to leave. I don't think any gym manager would argue with your decision here. But now you know this is an actual possibility, ask at the next opportunity.

Latecomers

This is always a touchy subject and unfortunately you need to go with the gym policy. As per any good group exercise programme certification, you should not have anyone join in after the warm-up is done.

In practical terms, if I know the person coming in late, and I know they can set up and warm up, I am fine with a little lateness. I also know that most seasoned riders would not try and join in halfway through the class.

If an unfamiliar face sneaks in, I am still able to determine if they are a total beginner as these will avoid eye contact with me and head right for the back of the room. As if them not looking at me meant that I can't see them.

If it is just a few minutes into the warm-up, I will get off the bike, approach them, set them up quickly while still leading the warm-up. I will ask them about injuries. If they clearly have never been on a bike before I will tell them off. Yes, some of you will frown at that but I need them to know that this is not something they should get into a habit of doing. Out of respect for other riders and for their own safety.

If it is more than 10 minutes since the class started, I will get the attention of the person walking in and signal to them that it is too late to join.

My recommendation is therefore to know the studio's policy but be reasonable in your approach.

If you allow someone in, they are your responsibility.

You cannot sit there with the attitude: 'Well, you came late, it's not my problem that you don't know how to set up or ride that damn bike. I don't care!'

I witnessed a situation like that when I was a class participant. The instructor rocked up five minutes late (!!!), mumbled something that sounded like 'any injuries?' without as much as a glance at the riders so even if someone put their hand up, she would not have seen it.

She started the class and another five minutes later a girl walked in and looked at the instructor with a questioning look of: 'can I still join in?' yet the instructor refused to acknowledge her. The girl happened to sit right next to me and it was apparent she had no idea even how to move the saddle up or down. I pointed to the levers trying to be helpful without getting off and getting too involved as I was just another rider in there. She then struggled to keep up and could not understand the resistance. All the time the instructor refused to acknowledge her.

Finally, I leaned towards the poor soul saying: 'If you can't keep up with the music, turn it to the left, even if the instructor keeps asking to go harder'. On seeing our exchange, the instructor got off her bike and approached the rider, first giving me daggers, and said very loudly: 'You come late to my class and now you are interrupting everyone by talking!' She then stormed off still giving the poor rider no direction. Yes, you heard that right. The instructor who was *late* berated a rider for being late, after allowing them to join the class.

Remember: you can't have it both ways. You let people in, you make it work by making sure that they are at least safe.

Headphones

It is a no-no. You come to a group exercise class you follow the class, which means you need to hear my instructions. It is first and foremost rude. Unless you simply want to use a free bike while the class is on and you have your own training plan, if you can find a remote corner where you will not confuse other riders by doing your own thing, help yourself.

That said, I have no problems with people riding to their own music is during the 20- or 60-minute FTP test. For that level of effort over such a long duration, every little helps. If you need heavy rock or metal music which I can guarantee you will not hear in my classes, bring your own.

If I spot someone with their headphones after we started the class, I will signal to them to take them out. If they do not follow, I will approach them and tell them that is a requirement that they must adhere to or they are more than welcome to use other bikes on the gym floor and ride to their own profile.

> **EXCEPTIONS:** there are exceptions to every rule. There is a girl in my class who always works super hard and follows the instructions, yet keeps her headphones in. That is because she has a brain injury and needs to minimise the noise. The headphones are not attached to anything and simply act as earplugs.

If noise levels are an issue and a rider uses ear plugs or headphones to lower it, I have no issue with that.

Cadence – excessively high or low

I my classes we keep RPM between 60–120. If a rider chooses to get their RPM higher and can do it with good form, I will not have an issue with it, but I still haven't seen it (apart from 10–15 sec all out sprints with sufficient resistance). If I have advanced riders who ride outdoors and want to tackle 55RPM and can do it without compromising their form, I have no issue with it. However, if they cannot handle it, I will call them out.

My pet peeve are latecomers who then proceed to ride in excess of 130RPM with no resistance bouncing madly all over the shop to 'speed up the warm-up'. Thankfully I only have one regular like that, but it takes all my strength not to strangle him. He's in his 70s and no amount of explaining is going to change his ways.

Riders doing their own thing

I believe that as an instructor you provide a structured group exercise workout that the group should follow. You are a qualified professional who knows what and why they ask of their riders. You know the correct way to set up the bike and the science that goes behind the workout you create.

What if they don't follow? This issue is two-fold. First, there is the case of contraindicated movements (riders performing moves you don't) and second, there are the riders who don't seem to be doing much for the duration.

I don't believe in the approach: 'it's their workout, let them do whatever they want as long as they are moving', but … Read on because as usual nothing is just black and white.

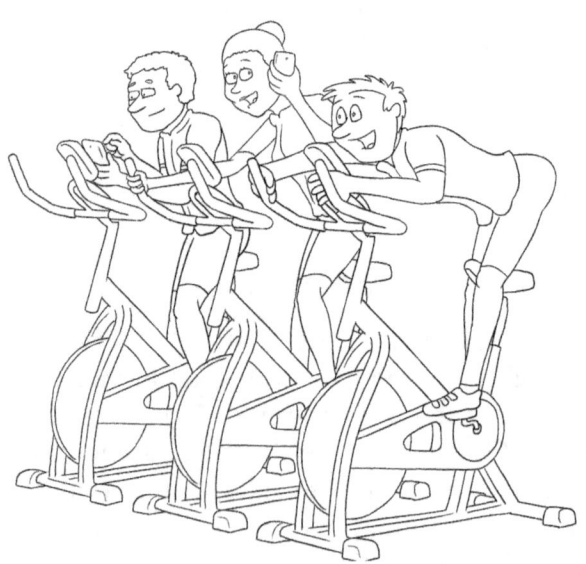

Contraindications

I talk more about it in the chapter *Keeping It Real*, but I teach what is known as the 'traditional' way or what I call 'no frills' way: no press ups, squats, tap backs or hovers etc. And as I consider these moves inefficient when performed on a bike but mainly unsafe, I do not tolerate them and will ask the riders to refrain from doing them.

Those who just plod along

These days many instructors say that since you don't know what is going on in people's lives you should let the participants do what they want. I disagree. I want to make sure that everyone gets the best out of each class and to do that I need to know why they are doing or not doing a certain move.

Therefore, before we start, I ask multiple times about injuries, offer help with the set up etc. I always give options for extra recoveries or to do the whole class seated even if I cue standing. If a rider tells me before the class that for whatever reason they will be taking it easy, I have no problem with that. If I am not aware of any mitigating circumstances, then I will most probably approach them at some point during the class to work out why they are not following the instructions.

How rigid should you be in this approach?

Do you confront these riders full on, all guns blazing? Are they just lazy? Let me tell you three stories that should help you decide on your approach.

Story #1 Numbers are my enemy

I teach using the coach by colour system on IC7s a lot. I do not have a problem with someone not using the colours, as long as they find the right intensity following my cues using the RPE scale, but usually after a couple of classes not using the colours, the riders do set the console up.

One girl after coming to the classes for a few months still would not put the colours on, yet would work extremely hard, always getting the intensity right as far as I could see from her body's response. Then she did her first 20 minutes FTP test. At the end of the FTP she said this was undoubtedly the hardest thing she had ever done and thanked me for my help and motivation. Still she would not set the colours up but still worked as hard as she could. I told her she was now definitely ready to start using the system but what she said in response was both surprising and thought provoking.

She had suffered from an eating disorder in the past when she was obsessed with numbers: calories, weight etc so she didn't want to get too number focused again, checking the percentages and averages as she was worried it could be a slippery slope in her recovery. The basic screen set up allowed her to monitor her cadence and resistance, so she would know she was maintaining whatever effort she was supposed to but still preferred listening to her body than chasing numbers.

The second story really touched my heart.

Story #2 Facing adversities

I had a lady in my class who was a regular. I noticed her because she would always meticulously clean her bike before getting on it (using two hand towels drenched in antibacterial gel). I did approach her in a couple of classes trying to get her to increase her effort as it looked like she was sticking to lower intensities than what I was trying to get her to achieve. She never looked bored or distracted though, so after making my point I just let her do her thing.

One week she came up to me before the start of the class and said she had taken a fall down the stairs in the morning and her bum and lower back were sore, but she decided to still give it a go. I told her that if it felt too uncomfortable, she was free to leave at any point.

As it turned out, she stayed for the full 45 minutes and she did most of it in the saddle. She was very focused, and I loved her determination. I did not get a chance to talk to her after the class as someone had approached me with a question and she left as I was talking to them.

I went into the changing rooms and as I was picking up my towels, still in my sweaty gear, I saw her ready to go into a shower. I went up to her to say well done and ask her about the back pain. She showed me a bruise on her arm from the fall and said that she was determined to get her workout in as keeping fit was her priority.

She then said she had been in remission from a rare form of leukaemia for over a year! That's why sometimes her watts may not look impressive (as she is still building back her strength after years of living with fatigue even before she got her diagnosis) but her heart rate responds the right way and she always gets the best she can out of the class even though she may not look like it. And that is also why she cleans her bike so religiously …

We then chatted away – me still in the sweaty gear, her in her towel – comparing notes on going through cancer and dealing with the process. We didn't even sit down because we were just having a quick chat.

Next, I looked at the clock and it was 9pm: we stood and talked for two hours! This woman's story should be made into a movie. She is a freaking superhero! And part of her keeping her sanity through the battle with cancer was attending indoor cycling classes regularly but being aware of her own limits and accepting them.

This story is another reminder that the first impressions we get of a person – and let's not kid ourselves, we all form an immediate judgement of a person in front of us – can be far from the truth. I could have marked her forever as an eccentric, cleaning-freak always trying to prove that she doesn't need me to be there. I am glad I didn't.

Final story is the most recent and one that was a big eye opener for me.

Story #3 Let me be

If you have been teaching for a long time you will have seen this on numerous occasions; those people who come to your classes and seemingly pay no attention to your instructions, take no notice of their bike setup, and just seem to plod along looking miserable. It's hard to not see them or not to get irritated.

I love teaching indoor cycling and I give 100 percent every time I stand in front of my riders. I will do my utmost to ensure that every person in that studio gets the best out of those 45 minutes. I go through bike setup every class, I structure my sessions well, I give clear targets at the start, and do my best to use various ways of motivating and conveying the intensity levels throughout the class.

If I see that someone is not following my instructions, I assume they struggle to understand what I want them to do. I will seek eye-to-eye contact with them to guide them and if that fails, I will approach them for a bit of one-on-one coaching.

While people are filing into the studio, I have made it a habit to announce that if anyone needs to take it easy for whatever reason, like an injury, to let me know so I will leave them in peace. People do take me up on it.

I would, however, get really wound up by riders who just walk in, usually last minute, plop on any bike without even checking if the brackets are locked, with complete disregard for the setup guidelines, and proceed to do a *big fat nothing* in terms of a workout for the duration of the class.

As an instructor, I would always feel conflicted when such a repeat offender would come in. On one hand, my professional conscience is clear since I have tried educating them and helping them out, yet they decide to ignore my suggestions and instructions and *still* turn up like clockwork. Should I ignore them completely and after four or five classes not even bother adjusting their bikes again? Is that ethical to just let them be? Should I even waste my breath and thought on riders like these? They clearly don't care!

I discussed this subject with a few fellow instructors and even some riders, and the consensus was that you can lead a horse to water, but you can't make it drink, so I should not worry myself with them. By ignoring me, *they* are being rude and so I should ignore them and focus on the rest of the group. It didn't sit well with me, but I decided to test my new approach and pretend I didn't see them in my next class.

Then one day, I was listening to a brilliant podcast called *Fitness Career Mastery*, episode 93 on how to motivate class participants and the do's and don'ts of group ex instructing.

One of the things talked about was that as important as motivation is in group exercise classes, it's equally important to acknowledge that some people just want to have some time away from their hectic office or personal life schedule and the intensity of the workout is not important to them. They mentioned an example of a yoga instructor who would say at the start of her class that if the participants wanted to stay in child's pose for the full hour, she was fine with that.

That took me slightly by surprise, but it was real food for thought. This is not something I would even think of doing as a participant, so it was hard for me to get my head around it. The crux of this approach was that if I, as an instructor, ask the riders to acknowledge their reason for coming in and that reason turns out to be simply escaping whatever else is happening in their lives, then they accomplish their goal by just being there. I shouldn't add to their stress by trying to make them work harder, albeit with good intentions, or tell them that by going easy they are wasting their time or even worse ... failing.

To be honest, this went against my instincts as an instructor, but it made me wonder if I had it all wrong.

Coincidentally, two days later I was covering a class in a facility where I have two such seemingly apathetic riders. I saw a woman walk in with a double buggy with a baby and a toddler. She smiled at me and I thought her face looked familiar, but I was struggling to work out where I knew her from. She then pointed to the buggy and said: 'This is the reason why I am always late to your class and why I have to rush off at the end. And it's why I cannot work any harder—I am totally exhausted!'

Only then did I realise that she was one of *those* two riders! I never got a chance to talk to her before or after the class, she always avoided eye contact during the class, and I have never ever seen her smile before! I suddenly felt so bad for thinking she was being rude, obstinate, or just could not be bothered.

From that moment on, I have been making a conscious effort in groups where I have riders like that, or if I notice someone who fits the bill, to say something along the lines of the following: "I want you to think about why you came into the studio today. What is your reason? Is it to get a great workout? Is it to work on improving your FTP? Is it to sweat off the stressful week in the office? Or is it simply the only 45 minutes in a week that you are free from your kids and responsibilities? If this is your 45 minutes of freedom and you want to take it easy—please do. I only ask you that you relax and enjoy it, maybe give me a smile from time to time so I know that you are doing it your way for the whole 45 minutes is a choice and not a result of you not understanding what I am asking of you. If this is your escape, I got you!'

The first time I said that, there was a great vibe and energy in the room as if people found this message refreshing, and some took me up on that offer, but they felt free to do that without trying to hide from me.

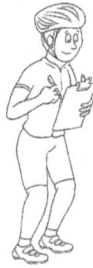

TACKLING STRATEGY: My take-away? As an instructor, it is important to notice individuals in your classes. Yes, it is hard when you have 30–40 people in the room. I struggle remembering names, I really suck at that. But I will remember the rider's injury or that they are preparing for a competition or what FTP we put in their bike last week.

Try and develop a rapport with your regulars so they feel they can come and talk to you. It can be done by arriving to the studio early so you can chat with people as they come in or staying behind for an extra few minutes after the class has finished so people can come and ask questions.

Do not be fixated on everyone doing the same thing every single second. Yes, it looks cool, but it is not necessary. Allow certain level of freedom so people take responsibility for their own workout. If they are respectful towards you and other riders in the room, let them ride seated for the whole class.

> 'People will not remember how much you knew but they will remember how much you cared'.

CHAPTER 5
Instructors' Dilemmas

To talk or not to talk? When to talk and what about.

This is one of the biggest dilemmas of an indoor cycling instructor. And it can be most controversial, right next to what kind of music you play. Know that the more nervous you are the more you will talk. Just like on a date ...

What needs to be said

Introduction
First, always introduce yourself. Every single time. Make it automatic. There will always be a new face in your class and it's just polite.

Class Duration
Remind the riders how long the class is. I always start by saying: 'I am Izabela and we have 45 minutes'. Some people may not know that your class is as long or short as it is. If a rider thinks a class is 45 minutes and then as they are ready to cool down there is no end in sight, it can be very confusing and frustrating. And sometimes when you cover a class you may think it's 45min but as soon as you say: 'The ride is 45 minutes' the people will shout back: 'No, it is 60 minutes actually'. Better to learn it at the start.

Goals
Either before you even start or in the early stages of a warm-up make sure you briefly explain the class goals. Say how many rounds of intervals are coming and how long they will be. Mention what intensities are to be expected etc. Leave details for later but say whether it's an endurance ride or sprint intervals. Is there a goal of achieving 'X' number of kilometres by the end of the class? Maybe an average power per class? Use something that you can check at the end so people can assess whether they have accomplished the mission.

Form

The fact that someone is watching the riders and can appraise their form makes the difference between taking a virtual class or riding on their own and an instructor-led workout. Therefore, watch your riders and mention what needs to be mentioned as and when you see it.

If everyone has their shoulders relaxed there is no need to mention it again. If you repeat the cue but the people who need to listen don't seem to, try saying it in a different way and accompany the words with an exaggerated movement: show them what you mean.

Intensity

These days many of us are lucky to ride high tech bikes with power meters or coach by colour system. I love using technology, yet I am fully aware that riding using colours (which represent power zones) only works if the correct FTP (functional threshold power) value has been entered. In short, if the person didn't set the gizmo right, the colours will represent just that – pretty colours with no meaning behind them. Therefore, using a very descriptive and *consistent* RPE (rate of perceived exertion) scale is key even with all that high tech.

What works for me is to give RPM range, explain the intensity by describing the feeling in the legs, breathing, etc., and then giving it a colour that this intensity corresponds with. I then add a caveat: 'If your RPM is what I asked for and the feeling is exactly what I asked for yet the colour is off, ignore the colour but make a mental note whether next time we need to increase your predicted FTP or take it down'.

Can I be silent?

Yes, yes you can! Is it easy? Hell, no! Despite seven years of experience and thousands of classes taught I still need to give myself permission to be silent as the basic instinct is to talk. When I say nothing for a while, nagging thoughts invade my head:

> *What am I doing here if I am not saying anything? Will they think I don't care?*

THEY WILL BE FINE, provided you explained what you wanted them to do. Sometimes people just want to focus on their effort and their workout. If your music is getting them into the zone, the last thing they want to hear if your incessant talk.

When to be silent?
When a song has got loads of lyrics, talking over the singer is awful from the riders' perspective, and it makes what you are saying unintelligible. If you don't think so I would recommend taking a couple of classes as a participant and you will change your mind.

Make sure you choose your moment with respect to the song played. When the lyrics already have a message, don't spoil it by talking over it.

When you want people to focus on something like their technique or pedal stroke. Explain the task and just let them ride in peace.

Do I just get off the grid?
If you know you are a talker and you are planning to work on it by going silent for two or three minutes, let the riders know. For example: "Next song is a six-minute hill. We will start together, find the rhythm and intensity. I will then let you go on your own. Next you will hear from me will be one minute from the top'.

How to be silent?
Boy oh boy. Not as easy as you think! You may need to switch the microphone off, to avoid temptation. Look at the timer and keep repeating in your head: *I can do this. I am strong. I've got this!*

You know, the same thing you tell your riders to do when they struggle with a challenge.

What to do when you are silent
You can do so much. You can observe the riders from your bike. You can still give out visual cues of relaxing the grip, knees position, relaxing the shoulders etc. You can catch eye contact with individual riders and give them the thumbs up. You can show someone clearly struggling that they can ease off and take a break just by using your face and gestures so nobody else even notices.

This is a perfect time to get off the bike and give people some one-to-one attention. See the chapter on teaching off the bike for more advice. I also use this time to go and refill people's water bottles if needed.

How do I know if I talk too much?
A very cringeworthy method of finding out is recording yourself. But then you must listen to it, and it may hurt.

If you consciously set out on a mission of reducing the amount of your talking, every time you are about to say something, stop and think: is it necessary? Haven't you just said it?

The method I use is to do an annual feedback form that I give out in my classes. (see Chapter 11 Feedback Forms). One question there is about the amount of talking I do: Do I talk too much or not enough? (Another one is: What is my catchphrase? Invaluable.)

How to say what you need to say?
This is quite a complex issue and it will come with experience. Using different tone of voice, visualisation techniques, adding jokes or stories, involving your riders, is what makes you YOU, and makes you stand out (see Chapter 10 on Teaching Styles) Learning how to use music when you talk is a great skill that comes with experience.

Turn the music down
Sometimes, to make sure nobody misses an important message, it helps to turn the music down a notch to ensure everyone's attention is on what you say.

Don't force it
… Whatever your natural style is, don't force yourself to talk as much or as little as another instructor. Yes, try things for measure but what works for them may not be suited to your personality. Just do you but remain open to constructive criticism and feedback. I guarantee that your style will evolve over the years.

Written notes – to script or not to script?

Some instructors, especially recently qualified ones, write down detailed notes of *everything* they want to say and how they want to say it. If it works for you, then do it. Sometimes your mind just goes blank so it's good to have a back-up.

There is no right or wrong option here. I have never heard a rider think less of an instructor for having notes.

There are a few important things to remember when you script *everything*. I talk about that in detail in Chapter 14 Using Notes.

Having a library of phrases, words describing intensity etc is something that you build over time.

How hard should I ride in class?

This is another point that often divides the indoor cycling instructors. Some say that they cannot demand from the riders what they cannot deliver themselves and strongly believe that the: 'look, I am with you all the way,' approach is what is a proof of whether they are a worthy instructor or not.

I will say it works for *some* instructors and it is what some riders love. One of the world-leading cycling programmes advises instructors to give 100 percent in all their classes as the only way to realise their true teaching potential. I beg to differ.

Do you need to know exactly what you are asking your riders to achieve? Yes. Should you be able to ride the profile yourself? Yes. Should you do it in every class? I believe not.

Whether this is currently your MO, or you think it should be, I will pose a couple of questions here for you to ponder before you decide if your current approach needs rethinking.

First, how many cycling classes do you teach in a day or week? If like many of us you do around 10 or even 15 every week, is it not an unreasonable expectation on behalf of your riders *and* yourself to give your 100 percent effort *to ride* each class as you want the participants to ride it? How many of them do the same volume as you do? If you teach many HIIT style classes, would you advise anyone to ride 10 of these a week?

Second, is your main job to prove to the riders your level of fitness or to ensure that you prepare and deliver a sound, structured class with clear goals with the rider in its centre of focus?

You will have seen the following phrase in many online forums: *It's not your workout!*

If I try to match my riders 100 percent (follow the class profile) I catch myself getting in the zone and becoming a rider as my focus shifts onto *my* numbers. I lose the eye contact with the riders and I am not fully aware what is going on in front of me. That is not desirable, not least from the point of view of safety.

My advice would be, *always* prioritise *your role in the room:* to deliver a group class, to be a teacher, a coach and an instructor. If you have insecurities and think that people will think less of you unless you go as hard as you want them to go, you need to address those. Why do you feel like that?

How to lead if not by example?

It may be more challenging for some instructors, but it can be beneficial for both sides. Think about different type of riders. Some are visual learners; others are more receptive to verbal cues. If you are working at threshold (or above) and your breathing reflects that making it at times impossible to give your cues clearly enough, is that going to be appreciated?

Use your body

What about the visual learners, I hear you say, they will want to copy me! But you can still use visual cues by using your hands, arms, legs and exaggerated moves to mimic relaxing shoulders/wrists/elbows, increase/decrease in resistance, focus, knees position, engaging your hamstrings, relaxing your face, increasing cadence etc. Be creative. Learn from other instructors and adapt what you like to create your style.

Get off the bike

This is a very helpful technique which I will discuss further in the next point.

Whatever your style, ask yourself this question: regardless of the size of your group, would you be able to say one thing about every single person in that class when it is finished? If any of them approached you with a question, would you even know which corner of the room they were sitting in? Trust me, this would be more appreciated than having watched *you* kill the workout on your bike.

WARNING! ALERT! WARNING! ALERT!

I have seen that too many times not to mention it. If you ride the whole class but choose to ride at a much lower intensity that your riders while *pretending* you are working as hard as them, you need to be aware of what you are asking people to do. Confused? Let me explain.

I rode in a class when an instructor was asking for 100RPM out of the saddle for one minute (impossible for most to achieve) while she was clearly riding around 70–80RPM. I saw another instructor ask for 'one more turn' for the seventh time, when they clearly have not even touched their resistance.

On IC7 bikes (where you can see the gear number you are on) I heard instructors yell out: 'Level 60!' (general population will probably not be able to go higher than high 40s for more than a handful of seconds) while they were happily bouncing around grinning at around level 30.

If there is one thing you will learn from reading this book, please make it be this:

> *If you are riding at a lower intensity than your riders,*
> *YOU NEED TO KNOW YOUR PROFILE INSIDE OUT so you*
> *know HOW YOU WOULD FEEL AT ANY POINT, WERE*
> *YOU RIDING IT AS PRESCRIBED!!!*

If you are not riding, use a profile you know inside out. Don't use a new profile you have just created but never tried. Particularly if your profiles are music driven (verse/chorus style). It's hard to work out if the recoveries are sufficient in this type of profile unless you try it.

When I used to build classes starting from the music and based solely on the changes within the songs, I would often create what

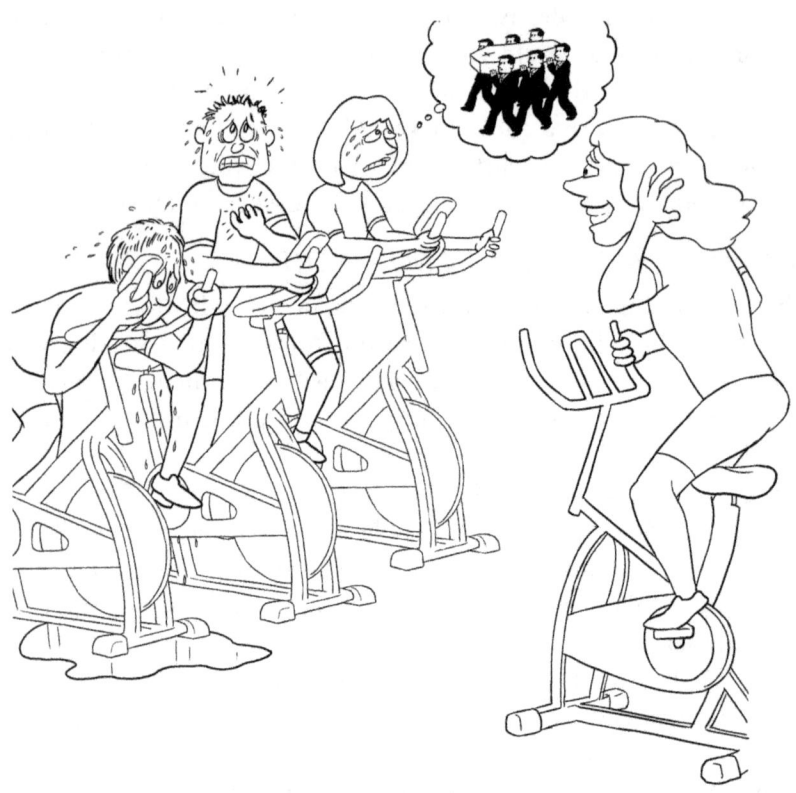

looked like an amazing profile on paper then get my class to ride it. Very often it would be clear that they weren't coping so I had to make ad hock changes moving recovery tracks around or asking for lower intensity efforts.

If you build your profiles based on power training zones and you understand work to recovery ratios (check Chapter 13 on Intensity), the risk of it happening is much lower. I try riding new profiles on my own before I teach them, but I also am in a great position when the first class of the week I teach is on IC7 bikes with the coach by colour system and the Connect system (big screen with data for all to see, including the group performance stats). The group is not too big, and they have been riding with me for years and with all the data and visuals they have I can take a step back and keep up with the profile 100 percent to have a feel of it.

On or off the bike?

This is another one of the most controversial topics. Just like with using notes, there is no right or wrong here. It either suits your style and personality, or it does not. If you teach on the bike 100 percent of the time, it does not make you automatically a better or worse instructor from the ones who get off a couple of times or teach completely off the bike.

I have been a strong advocate of the opinion that teaching on and off the bike are two very different styles. Teaching from the floor will not suit every instructor or be accepted by every group of riders, or even studio managers. Some instructors do not get off, but stop pedalling when they focus on coaching.

Why you may want to stay on the bike the whole time

- VISIBILITY – especially if your bike is on a podium, it makes it easier for you to see the riders and for them to see you.
- LIGHTS AND MUSIC CONTROLS – these are normally at your fingertips when you are on the instructor's bike.
- YOU LIKE TO LEAD BY EXAMPLE – you are of the opinion that you should do exactly what you are asking of your riders.
- YOU WANT TO MAKE THE RIDERS FEEL YOU'RE A TEAM – 'I am with you! Look, we are suffering the same fate here'.
- YOU ARE A RELATIVELY NEW INSTRUCTOR and teaching off the bike requires experience and confidence as well as knowing your class profile inside out, so you don't need to see your phone screen or notes to know what is coming next.
- THIS IS A SKILL YOU HAVE TO STILL AQUIRE and it is hard to break with the habit of always being on the bike so despite saying to yourself you will try it; you end up teaching your usual way every time.

... Why you may want to get off the bike (for a bit) or teach the whole class off the bike

- YOU HAVE AN INJURY – this is how most instructors get introduced to teaching from the floor: they cannot ride. In this scenario this skill is invaluable if you do not want to lose income.
- YOU HAVE A BIG GROUP OF RIDERS (over 30) AND WANT TO GIVE THEM INDIVIDUAL ATTENTION – in a studio that big, most of the time anyone past row four cannot see you anyway, they simply copy the person in front of them. Walking around helps you connect to your riders and give specific corrections or praise. You also get to connect with those who never give you eye contact when you are on your bike.
- YOU WANT TO CHALLENGE YOURSELF AS AN INSTRUCTOR – can you cue and motivate people just by your voice and using gestures? It forces you to expand your instructor toolbox.
- YOU WANT TO EMPOWER YOUR RIDERS BY TEACHING THEM INTRINSIC MOTIVATION – if you ask your riders open questions, give them choices, ask them to remember why they are on that bike, you help them learn to take responsibility for their own workout. When they know their WHY, they do not need to see you pedal, to get motivated.
- IF YOU ARE A TALKER – when you walk around giving one-to-one you do it off the mic so the other riders get a break from your talking and can just get in the zone which works particularly well on long tracks 7–15 minutes long.
- IF YOUR CLASS IS FULL – and an extra rider turns up. I will discuss it further in the next point.

So, there you have it. It's undoubtedly an incredibly useful skill to have but if it is not *you*, then don't force it. If you however like to challenge yourself as an instructor, then try it.

Giving up your bike

This is very closely connected to the previous point as for you to be able to give up your bike, you need the skill of teaching off the bike. The circumstances may be that the class is fully booked or overbooked as one of the bikes is faulty and cannot be used.

I would be inclined to state that the less experience you have as a group exercise instructor, the more you *need* your bike. Just like a budding singer needs his guitar or a piano to feel comfortable on stage; they are good but take their instrument away and their confidence plummets, their body becomes rigid and they don't know what to do with their hands. Practice makes perfect though.

The question is then, should you give up your own bike?

If you are only covering in a studio you don't know much about, I would be cautious. Maybe even ask the studio manager first. The riders may have not ridden a class like that before, and the management may not be too happy about that.

If it's your regular class and the riders are used to you not riding all the time, I promise you they will not bat an eyelid. The challenge may be finding a rider that is willing to take your bike, especially if it's positioned on a stand and visible to all. It can be really intimidating. Many times, there were no takers despite me offering it. However, those who did put their hand up always said to me at the end that they were too busy working hard to be bothered about whether people were watching them and when they did look at the group, nobody seemed to pay much attention to them anyway.

The same rule applies that I have already mentioned above: *know what you are asking for.*

How Many Classes is too Many?

Many instructors ask on various forums about what number of classes others teach a week. There is no universal limit that would apply to all. All depends on your workload (as in your daytime job), family life, other commitments, fitness level, etc. There are people teaching 20–30 classes a week but those often include private clients or other formats like circuits or yoga etc.

My personal stand on this based on experience is that your body can get used to *anything*. I started teaching classes working full time 9–5:30pm Monday to Friday doing an office job. I was teaching early mornings, some lunchtimes, evenings and weekends. I started from 3–4 a week and ended up on 14 indoor cycling classes a week on top of my office job. Yes, I was younger but looking back I still don't understand how I did it.

Why did I decide to reduce the number? I was getting into a state of accumulated fatigue where my legs were permanently stiff, my back was achy, my feet were rigid, and I didn't even have time to go and get a massage. Then I started getting snappy with my riders. I had no patience when people were not following instructions. I even got as far as turning someone's resistance up for them quite drastically – I am not proud of that – and that's when I knew it was too much. Teaching has become just another job that I was too tired to do properly.

I reduced the number of one-off classes and started to teach off the bike more just to save my body and focus more on what I consider my main role when I am in front of any group of riders in a studio – instructing.

I only teach indoor cycling, no other formats so it's a bit harder. Ideal situation would be combining indoor cycling with swimming or yoga or Pilates. I currently have nine fixed classes a week and I work part-time as an accountant. I found my happy medium.

Do not feel pressured when someone teaches double what you do or think that your body will cope with it because someone else's has. Or think you need to give up some classes simply because someone said it's too many.

If you are still happy to wake up at 5am for your morning class, if despite years of teaching you are still passionate about creating new profiles and feel pride when your riders improve, start taking part in outdoor competitions or even train as instructors themselves, then keep doing what you are doing.

If you feel burnt out and start questioning why you are still doing it, then take the foot off the gas or take a complete break.

I know we are not maths or science teachers, but the same

principle applies. If your face and body language say you don't really want to do this, this is exactly what people will pick up on. You need to keep the passion alive. I talk about how to do this in Chapter 15 on Motivation.

CHAPTER 6
Class Profiles

This chapter will give you a general idea on how to create a class profile and what platform to use. It would take a separate book to discuss it in detail and still nothing could replace actual practice.

If you are a Les Mills RPM (or other format) instructor, you don't have to worry about this issue as the profile and the accompanying music is given to you. However, I have seen posts from LM instructors who decide to go freestyle and feel really lost and do not know where to start building their own class.

Chicken or the egg? Music or profile first?

My original qualification was with YMCA and Keiser, but I must say I knew nothing about creating a class profile at the end of that one-day course. If you are a freshly qualified instructor who shares this feeling and doesn't teach with power, then my advice would be start from the music and use the changes in tempo or beat to drive the class.

I see many seasoned instructors frowning at this suggestion and I can almost hear what you are saying now: 'No! Get into the right habit from the start and always have a profile in mind first!' Trust me, I see your point. This is how I create my classes *now* as well; however, when you feel lost, overwhelmed and don't have ideas for a profile, you start from your strengths by using your favourite songs and just go with the flow of the music. Get your bearings and build your confidence this way. All the while research forums, try apps for profiles which you can then add your music to before you feel confident enough to start creating your own from scratch.

Things to remember

When creating your own profile, the basics you need to consider are:

Who are your riders?

What is the population? Mainly regulars? Always new people? Can you build on the previous class? Are they rhythm riders or do many ride outdoors? Will they appreciate long 8–10-minute intervals, or will they not be able to focus for that long?

How long is the class?

This will determine the length of your warm-up (and its intensity) and cool-down. Your warm-up for 45-minute class will be shorter than for a 90-minute one. Same with the cool-down.

What you do in the warm-up will be dictated by what comes after. Will it be steady state long intervals? Will it be HIT?

Do people come on time?

It may sound like a weird question, but I teach in places where people come in 20 minutes early and I can really start early as everyone is ready to go five minutes ahead of schedule. Then there is this place where every week people come on the dot or a couple of minutes late. I cannot keep them for extra five minutes as there is another class straight after, so I need to plan for five minutes less.

What is the purpose/goal of your class?

This may be simply to have fun and sing along, get used to staying in the saddle for long periods, working on muscular strength, working on maximum power intervals etc. Ideally, your purpose should come before the music.

Where do I put the recoveries?

Look up Chapter 13 on intensity to learn more about recoveries.

Profile resources and building platforms

You can also get fantastic profiles from some of the Facebook forums and the ICA (Indoor Cycling Association). Try and use recommended sites or apps and be cautious when you just come across a random website or a YouTube video. There are plenty of rogue profiles in the ether that claim to be bees' knees, when in fact they are completely unrealistic.

Acronyms in profiles

If you find a profile online, you may see these acronyms in them:

RPM – revolutions per minute.
FTP – functional threshold power.
FTW – functional threshold wattage.
WI – work interval.
RBI – rest between intervals.
NP – normalised power.
STC – standing or seated climb.
IF – intensity factor (worth reading up on if you teach on Lifetime Fitness IC6 or IC7 bikes).
TSS – training stress score (worth reading up on if you teach on Lifetime Fitness IC6 or IC7 bikes).
Z1-Z5 (or up to Z7) – power zones which go from 1–5 or 1–7 depending on the bike/data console used.

Where to find good quality profiles?

As mentioned above, ICA has a vast library of class profiles with accompanying playlists and detailed class notes available to its members. I would recommend joining them.

You can follow some instructors on Spotify to get playlists with interesting music and then build your own profile around them.

Cycling Fusion has an app **Class Builder** where you can build profiles using power zones.

If you are a **Stages** instructor, you can use their online platform Stages Flight to create profiles and use existing profiles from the database. These are based on the seven power zones, so you need your knowledge of teaching with power to understand these profiles and to be able to spot bad ones.

If you teach on Life Fitness bikes IC8, IC7 or IC6 with Coach by Colour system, you can use **ICG Training app** which has quite a few profiles built in and where you can create, exchange/share profiles with other instructors.

There is a great app called **Intelligent Cycling** with numerous profiles arranged by categories and using the power zones and colours system. These are linked to ready-made Spotify playlists. This platform is super user-friendly when it comes to creating your own profiles. You can switch between various colour zone systems used by different bikes (Stages vs Life Fitness). You can build your own library of profiles, you can swap and share with other instructors and your riders can use these profiles as well.

There is the **Sufferfest** app with profiles, music and visuals to match but their profiles are often too advanced for a general population. You can always adapt them to your needs.

Finally, you can get your inspiration from using systems like **Zwift**, **Peloton**. You can look at training programmes on Wattbike or British Cycling websites to help you create your own class profiles.

There are other apps on the market, too. You just need to find what suits you best.

But How Do I Create My Own?

> DISCLAIMER: before you create your own profile (or borrow one) using power zones you must have a good understanding of what these power zones mean in terms of intensity and how long an average gym goer is able to work in each. Not every profile out there is worth using or even should be used! Ask someone with experience for feedback.

When creating a new profile or deciding on a profile you will use, a few simple steps apply:

- **How long** is the class? Based on that leave appropriate time for **warm-up** and **cool-down**.

- What is the **goal** of the class? Is it VO2max intervals/sprints/Z3 long intervals/continuous ride/staying in the saddle as long as possible/FTP test?
- Remember that **LESS IS MORE**.
- Apply the appropriate **work to rest ratios** THIS IS CRUCIAL AND A BASE OF EVERY GOOD PROFILE! Below you will find the ratios as recommended by Stages Cycling.

INTERVAL TYPE	MINIMUM	MAXIMUM
Aerobic intervals (Z3–Z4)	2:1	4:1
VO2 max (Z5)	1:1	1:2
Anaerobic (Z6)	1:3	1:4
Neuromuscular Power (Z7)	1:4	1:8

- Find the right music.
- Ride it.
- Tweak it (if needed).
- Use it in class.
- Tweak it (if needed).
- Save for future use.

A word of advice, when it comes to saving a profile as a Spotify or iTunes playlist: put as many details as you can in the title unless you keep a file of notes that has a reference to a specific playlist. Many times, I created a great profile, practised it in my head, used it in classes but then a few months later could not remember what I did with that playlist!

Having learnt my lesson, if a profile is music driven, I will name it something like '7m hill/14m flat/8x30sec max'. If it is a very specific interval ride using power zones, my titles are so long that you cannot see the entire ones at times, but it's always easy to work out the exact structure even a year down the line.

Another option is to give a profile a name like Killer 2019 or Hot Gates or Boiling Frogs and then write notes on the exact structure in your notes app on the phone or in an email. I take a screen shot of the playlist and the notes and e-mail these to myself with the title of the class in the subject. This way even if I change phones or lose a playlist, I can recreate it. Find a way that works for you. Also check out Chapter 8 on Music for further advice.

Progressive Profiles

If you write or use a very structured profile, it may be worth developing into a series of four or even six. You may increase the number of intervals each week, their length or intensity or shorten the recoveries. Just keep the PURPOSE and work to rest ratio in mind and world is your oyster.

CHAPTER 7

Music

What Medium to Use?

I live and work in the UK where everything used to be much clearer a few years back in terms of music licensing. Instructors had to buy their own PPL licence and gyms had to buy theirs. It was a one-off annual fee for us, and we were good to go.

Then they made things 'easier' and instructors were no longer required to buy the PPL licence with the burden being put totally on the gyms and studios. Individuals only need a PPL licence if they teach in venues like church halls etc.

Consequently, some gyms started charging instructors to recuperate the costs by deducting a fee for each class taught using licenced (original) music. To illustrate: if the rate is £25 per class, they would now pay £23.70 unless instructors declared that they only played PPL free music.

The PPL free music can be purchased from various sites and is generally (in my opinion) quite awful unless you are a DJ or a person skilled in using Mix Meister and can create your own mixes.

I have built up my library of playlists using iTunes. I paid for the songs. The studios I teach at pay for the right to play them, so all is fair and square.

Spotify

As of writing this book, all the research I have done states that using Spotify in gym classes in the UK (even if you have the premium licence) is fuzzy grey. Even if the gym pays a fee to the licensing agency to stream music, if you have a personal Spotify licence you are in breach of your contract with Spotify.

Spotify Business is a commercial licence that does allow you to stream in a business environment so please check with your gym or studio. If the gym's licence is in order you have nothing to fear from the licencing body but can still be sued by Spotify if using personal licence.

Certain gyms specifically prohibit streaming music in classes so check with the management before taking a new class on.

Your device

We tend to use our phones for everything, but I still use an iPad for my music. Many people use their laptops or iMacs (the Mix Meister users). I have auditioned for a chain where they would not allow using your phone to play music claiming the sound quality is not as good as when using an iPad or a laptop.

What type of Music to Use?

This is where your personality comes into play. You as an instructor must enjoy the music you play. If you decide to play a whole class of rock music only because John on Tuesdays always plays rock and his classes are full, you may discover it doesn't work for you (if deep down you cannot stand rock as your face will betray you).

If your riders request a certain genre that is not your thing, you can play a song or two here or there but do not feel bullied into submission.

If you decide to borrow a profile from someone and it comes with a playlist, listen to it from top to bottom and decide if it suits you. I borrowed many profiles from many great instructors but when I tried to do the same with the accompanying playlists, I felt like I wanted to slash my wrists. I have no doubt the playlists worked perfectly for people who created them, but I couldn't connect with the songs.

That is not to say that you shouldn't challenge yourself from time to time and use a track that will get you out of your comfort zone. I love using classical music, film scores, even old school swing.

I have a couple of playlists in my library called Across the Music. I always introduce this profile by saying:

> *Today's class is very much music driven. If you like a song, enjoy it because the next one will be a different genre. If you don't like a song, don't worry because the next one will be a different genre."*

One of them has Irish Lord of the Dance track, Prodigy, Elton John, Michael Jackson, and Mack the Knife by Bublé …

I also have a profile which is a very precise interval ride of 30/60/30/120 seconds for nine rounds but since I am not a DJ and I do not mix my own music I simply use a continuous dance mix from one of the Tomorrowland mixes. Yes, the beat changes here and there but it does not matter as the task at hand is clear and the timer is on. Music simply provides a background to disguise the heavy breathing.

What Not to Use?

Swearing

Be careful of swearwords. One here or there is not a big deal and you can always try and talk over it but a song full of expletives may not be appreciated.

What about reggae, country or Latin?

Reggae music is not generally suitable for indoor cycling, but you can find a song that would work for a cool down or recovery.

Living in the UK I cannot comment on country music and I do not need to for that reason alone, but Keith Urban does feature in my classes.

My favourite music outside of gym is Latin with a capital L. I love Salsa. Unfortunately, it is totally unsuitable for indoor cycling as it is either too slow or too fast, but you can use the more commercial songs by Pitbull or JLO. Reggaeton songs can be used for slower climbs.

One-genre playlists

If you decide to play only rock for 45 minutes, it may be risky unless you know your audience well. Or if you go with just one artist for the whole session. If you as a rider happen to hate the genre or the artist, then you are about to suffer badly for 45 or 60 minutes.

In 2019 I created a well-received Tina Turner tribute playlist, a Roxette one and Rock Classics (AC/DC, Aerosmith, Scorpions, Bruce Springsteen, ZZ Top).

Useful advice

Try and use tracks with not too many lyrics or just instrumental as your first song so you can explain the class profile and talk about the goals etc without having to compete with the singer.

Motivational Speeches

I came across this concept on an instructor forum. I like experimenting and challenging myself, but you also need to know your audience. I use one song which uses parts of Martin Luther King's 'I have a Dream' speech, but it is built into the melody, so it is not the raw speech itself.

I have bought a whole album of short motivational speeches, about 1–2 minutes long, that I use in my 20- and 60-minute FTP test playlists.

X versus Y playlists and Theme Rides

These are like Marmite – you either love them or hate them. I believe that if you can still have a clear goal for your ride and can make a playlist of two artists only work for you, that's great. I myself have a playlist called John Newman intervals. He has sung, or featured in, enough songs for a whole playlist, and they are all nice, and short, so it works like a charm.

When it comes to themed rides, I love **TDF** (Tour de France) profiles where I use an actual TDF profile adapted to my class, decorate the room with flags and TDF posters and use a lot of Kraftwerk music. I always do a **Halloween** themed ride complete with fancy dress and decorations, and a couple of times a year I ride the **Top Gun** profile (see ICA website).

Some instructors take a theme ride to another level using certain words like 'rain' or 'sun' or 'holiday' as their theme and using only songs with these words in titles. It is very time consuming, in my opinion, but again if that keeps your passion going, then go for it! As long as it does not take away from the purpose and effectiveness of the workout, knock yourself out. There can be a playlist for any occasion.

How Not to Spend Hours Creating Your Playlists?

Create your playlist around a profile

If you do that, you can build two or three versions of it so you can still use the same profile, but your riders may not even be aware of it. If you build your ride around the music where you stand up or sprint during the chorus, then there may not be much else you can do with it, and you can only ride it one way.

Pimp your existing playlists

If you create a playlist that you really like, but as time goes by it loses its relevance, create a version B and replace a song or two with something more current. Keep the original though as it may become one of those vintage playlists you go back to every year.

Use someone else's playlist

As mentioned before, you can follow people on Spotify or use resources like ICA website or Intelligent Cycling app where all profiles have an accompanying playlist attached.

But the key to saving your time is categorising whatever music and playlists you already have.

How to categorise your music

I have always used iTunes and even though I do have a Spotify account it's more for getting ideas for songs, therefore I can't give you any advice on categorising music on Spotify, but I will tell you what works for me in iTunes.

When I buy a song, I listen to it and decide if it is good for warm up, cool down, steady state or intervals. If it's intervals I will add the breakdown to the title, i.e. 15/15/30.

I will also get either its exact bpm or give a general range of fast 80–100RPM or 60–70RPM climb. I click on the song's info and enter the RPM and any useful comment like Warm up/cool down etc there.

In my iTunes library I added columns for BPM, which I use for RPM, and a Comments column which I use for categories of use.

When it comes to naming whole playlists, this is what works for me:

- Start with the duration: 30/45/60/90 minutes.
- Give it a name if it makes it obvious what the profile is about, i.e. LT Intervals 4x4 3RBI (lactate threshold intervals 4 x 4min, 3 minutes rest between intervals) or 15H/8F/15H (15 min hill, 8 min flat, 15 min hill).
- In time driven profiles the name can read 3 x (3x2@110% 1RBI) – 3 rounds of 3 x 2 min at 110% threshold with 1-minute rests between intervals; this description is detailed enough for me to be able to know what it's about at a glance.
- If I keep the same profile but create a new playlist for it, I may duplicate the title but add month and year at the and so I may have: 3 x (3x2@110% 1RBI) Jan17 & 3 x (3x2@110% 1RBI) Apr19.
- If I have a progressive profile that gets tougher every week, I will name it:

    45 Cadence Play 8m WUp/15s@125% 115RPM 2.45s@90% 85RPM W1. Read: 45 min ride with cadence drills as its purpose. 8 minutes warm up. Then 15 sec at 115RPM around 125% threshold followed by 2min 45s at 85RPM and 90% threshold.

    I will then look at the playlist to see what the length of work intervals was and what the RBIs were. There is a limit to what you can put into the playlist's title before it starts looking ridiculous.

CHAPTER 8

How to Put Bums on Seats and Keep Your Classes Busy

Be a Pro!

Attire

First and foremost, always be a professional and show respect for your riders by looking and acting like one.

By looking like a pro, I mean wear clean, fresh clothes and ideally cycling shoes. The kit doesn't have to consist of padded shorts and a cycling jersey. I find these items make me too hot indoors.

When I wear padded shorts indoors and get off the bike at the end of the class, the sweat from the padding starts running down my legs giving the impression of incontinence … And a zipped-up jersey makes me feel somewhat claustrophobic as many places I teach at don't have adequate air conditioning.

However, there is nothing wrong with you wearing outdoor cycling gear if you are comfortable in it. It makes you look like you know what you are doing and may tempt outdoor cyclists to try your class. By the same token this look may put off some newbies who may be intimidated by your kit but hey, you can't win them all.

Instructor's physique

This always causes controversy. Are riders or clients attracted to classes led by an instructor who looks like an Instagram model or to someone who looks more like them or maybe looks don't matter at all? After a discussion on this topic with a few fellow instructors, the views are divided. If we are selling our services telling people that attending our classes will keep them in shape, what if we don't look like we are?

Some people will want to have a super fit and beautiful person in front of them as a motivation to what they aspire to be. Others will appreciate someone who looks more 'accessible', like they would understand what Steve or Jane are going through trying to get in shape.

To me personally, if a female instructor rocks up with tons of make-up and long hair not in a pony tail, it immediately puts me on alert – are they going to make us work hard or is it one of those who make their image a priority? It is not always the case and I am not bashing anyone for liking make-up more than me, but this is my experience.

If an instructor spends the last few minutes before the start taking selfies from various angles (yep, I have seen that), I pass. It dehumanises them in my eyes. I feel intimidated and would not approach them to ask for help.

There are instructors out there of all shapes and sizes and all ages. Having ripped abs and big 'guns' doesn't make you a better instructor than someone who doesn't have clear muscle definition. I am more focused on instructors' knowledge, a well-structured class and the way they interact with the riders than on what size they are and this is true for many riders.

Punctuality

There is nothing worse than an instructor being late all the time or starting the class late all the time. Yes, I sometimes may start a minute or two late if I get late comers and I am setting them up, but I will endeavour to cue the warm up regardless whether I am on my bike or in the middle of the room adjusting someone's seat. And I am always in the studio at least 15 minutes before the start.

By the same token try not to overrun your classes as it is not fair on the riders who may have other commitments or another instructor who teaches directly after you and you taking two minutes longer than your allotted slot means that they have two minutes less to set up the room and their riders. Respect your colleagues.

Be prepared

Another sign of respect is always turning up prepared: kit, batteries etc. but first, class plan or profile. You should be able to say in a couple of sentences what the focus of the ride will be and to give a quick summary of its structure. This always makes you look like someone who takes their job seriously. I would never just put a playlist on shuffle and wing it start to finish out of choice (maybe in an emergency). Could I pull it off? Most probably. But it would make me feel like I lowered my standards.

Stand Out

Is there anything that makes you stand out as an instructor? Do you know what it is? If you don't know, start interacting with your riders before or after the class. Consider using social media to build a buzz around your classes and use them as motivation to bring people in. Know your audience.

Build a personal rapport with your regulars. Learn about their goals, injuries, work, etc. Running a business Facebook page or an Instagram account is great for that if people always seem to rush in and out of your early morning slot. This way they can comment or message you whenever.

It is also important to follow back the riders who follow you, to show you care and build a connection – like and comment on their posts and tag them in posts about the classes.

Do your best at learning riders' names even though this can be an immense challenge. For me it's an uphill battle. Unless someone follows me on social media or I manage to speak to them on a few occasions, their name will not stay in my head. But I will remember their FTP, or their injury, or that they wanted me to look at their set up next time they came, or the fact they were training for a half marathon.

Be known as the instructor who always checks everyone's bike set up and asks about injuries. My esteemed Stages Cycling colleague Glen was once asked by a rider: 'How do you determine if an instructor is good when you first take their class?'

His response was on point: *"Do they go through and check bike set up at the start of every class? If they don't, find another one."* (mic drop.)

Other things that make you unique may *become* your trademarks: your own music mixes, the fact that your music always matches the intervals to the second, or the fact that your class is structured in such a way and you are cueing in such a way that nobody even realises you play the same song three times in one class. It may be your unique sense of humour or your catchphrase.

Catchphrase? Don't you have one? Are you sure? Ask your riders. I didn't think I had one until I started doing feedback *forms* where one of the questions was asking about it. It turns out there are a few and here are my top three: 'Wiggle your toes', 'Do not waste your time', and 'If your console is red but your face is not, it's not because you are Bradley Wiggins, it's because you are cheating'.

Imitation is the best form of flattery – adopt or adapt?

One of the reasons you are reading this book is to learn how other instructor do things so you can learn and develop. We learn best by imitating others, but imitation can be a double-edged sword.

When you learn a new motivational quote or phrase or maybe a new way of explaining a concept that you heard from a Master *Instructor*, at the start you may simply copy it word for word when addressing your riders. But watch their reaction: do they seem to 'get it' as well as you did when you heard it? If yes, adopt it.

If not, you must adapt it. Was it the context or delivery that did not feel right? Maybe it was obvious the phrase did not come from you and you were just reciting a script? Make it sound like you and make sure it is relevant to your *audience*. It may be a slight change, or the phrase may no longer be recognisable. Either outcome is great if you have become a better instructor and your riders have benefited from it.

The one simple rule is that if you don't believe in what you are saying, neither will the riders. Be yourself.

Be yourself but dial it down if needed

Being yourself can carry a risk if it means being a loud drill sergeant who happens to swear a few times during a class and gets into people's faces. This may be exactly what your regular audience wants and enjoys, but it may be too much for a first timer to handle. They may feel intimidated and dread you approaching them. They may not know whether you are someone they can ask a question or whether you are just too militant in your approach.

Be mindful of how you come across. Make a point of approaching the new face beforehand with a smile so they see that side of you, too. Prewarn them by saying: 'This group enjoys being bossed around. Some of them are quite loud and you may hear a swearword when we go for the gut out effort.' Maybe give them a wink while you are at it. If they say this is what they are used to, you may include them in your usual banter and approach. Otherwise give them space while still acknowledging them in a milder manner or don't use any swear words at all. If you use songs with many rude words, it is also a good idea to prewarn any new riders.

Recognition Prizes

My pal and fellow Stages instructor Glen introduced me to the idea. To be exact, I saw this on his social media and 'stole' the idea from him (after a brief discussion about the details).

Glen introduced the Cycling Star award in his classes and got some awesome trophies on Amazon. They looked amazing, did not cost much and you could customise them with riders' names or names of categories.

I gave out a few of them in the following categories:

> Always Smiling Through Pain.
> Never Missing a Class.
> Best Spin Family (husband and wife sharing childcare so either one of them is always in my class).
> Best Back Row Crew (two friends who would come to all three morning classes and work their hardest at the very back of the studio).

I kept a few as special recognition prizes. One of them went to a guy who started taking my classes just a few weeks earlier. He came with no idea how to set up the bike or use the console and his cardio fitness was low. It was just his luck that his first class was our preparation for 20-minute FTP test so for the next two weeks he attended four sessions where we rode the 20-minute test. Not only was he not put off, but he got better results each time. He then continued to come three times a week and then brought his fiancé along.

His fitness improved so much, and his determination was so admirable, I gave him the award in recognition of just that. After the class he came to thank me and said that him and his fiancé were trying to get in shape for their upcoming wedding and that little trophy made him extremely happy and boosted his confidence and motivation.

They continued with my classes until their wedding day. When they returned from their nuptials, they continued until they moved to Australia. During their last week in the UK I was collecting donations for a charity close to my heart. At the end of their last class they approached me with a big carrier bag containing a massive glass jar full of coins they had been collecting for years. They offered it as their donation saying that my classes have touched their lives and they wanted to say thank you. I am welling up as I am writing this, but I was a blabbering mess at the time. It turned out to be quite a lot of money for which the charity was extremely grateful for (and didn't mind it took them two hours to count it). Thank you, Carlo and Chelsea!

I also decided to recognise a rider who is the strongest I have ever had in my classes. He is there front row and centre and despite his incredible fitness, he is always super friendly and humble.

But the main advantage of having him there is that he is the source of motivation for everyone else sitting in the front two rows. They all get a kick up their backside every class trying to push themselves that little extra because: if Morgan is killing it (and is about to keel over) I must give it my best!

If for whatever reason he is not there, I have people comment on my social media posts checking up on him. That's why as a thank you I got him a Superman cycling jersey and he got a round of applause from the group.

All these things: prizes, T-shirts etc. are your business expenses, so they are deductible from your tax bill, but they do not need to be super expensive. If you are creative, you can make some unique items. I remember Stages Cycling UK giving out cool recognition trophies made from bicycle parts.

Challenges and Games

Challenges

Over the years I have run three annual **Izabela's 50 Class Cycle SMART Challenges**. It starts on 1 November and finishes on the last day of February making it 150 days to complete 50 classes (three a week). There is an additional distance challenge where riders track their distances at the end of each class and strive to complete the distance of the epic ride from Land's End to John O'Groats. I use the mirror in the studio to keep the record of the rankings throughout the challenge.

I also use this challenge to encourage people to try different classes that may complement their fitness, like Pilates or yoga and do one of these a week for 150 days.

Participants also choose another measurable goal that may be able to do with their body weight (loose 5kg, lose X% of body fat) or not (run 10km without stopping, sign up and complete a 5km race, do 50 push ups without a break etc).

They are given a chart to track their progress but ultimately, *they are responsible for it*. There is no 'challenge police'. I also don't monopolise the challenge, meaning they do not even have to take *my* cycling classes (or even use a gym I work at), they can go to any class on the timetable.

Participants get weekly e-mails offering advice and updates on the results and sometimes suggesting extra short challenges within the main one.

They are then asked to review their progress and goals halfway through and modify them if needed. Christmas falls right bang in the middle of this challenge which is the biggest obstacle of all.

At the end, people send me their complete progress charts and feedback on their achievements, and I decide who gets to get a prize. I give out mugs and T-shirts with the logo of the challenge and the winners get good quality hoodies.

It is a lot of work mainly because of the duration but it is always a great success and I get lovely thank you e-mails and cards at the end. The reason for making it that long is that after 150 days you are more likely to stick to your new schedule and make it a part of your lifestyle than you would be after a week or two.

That said, there is nothing wrong with shorter challenges like trying to attend as many classes as possible in a week or a month. Or completing a distance or points challenge of some sort. You may do an FTP test in class, send riders a programme to follow in their own time, then retest in class after a set period, and reward the biggest improvements.

Sometimes simply running a challenge of completing a specific profile with the highest distance or average power or the highest maximum power at the end of that class is enough to motivate the riders. I then use the mirror and my social media to boast of people's success. Many won't be interested to have their name up there, but you would be surprised how many people thrive on that and challenge themselves extra hard to beat the competition. Just having your name up is their reward.

Games

Some instructors are good at these and have different ideas to make their classes more interactive using games like Trivia; however, I strongly believe this is more likely to work in America than in the UK. Due to the 'stiff upper lip' that the British are so famous for I even resort to cueing:

> *'Don't be British! Be vocal! You are now riding at 120–130 percent of your threshold. It HURTS. BAD. Shout, swear, scream if it helps. Don't hold it in. If it doesn't hurt – are you sure you are at nine out of 10 intensity?'*

You would be surprised how many riders let out an 'Aaaaargh!!!'" or 'C'mon!!! on hearing that.

By the same token relying on a game when your riders must answer questions, make suggestions or communicate with one another in order to keep the class going, is likely to flop miserably in the UK.

There is nothing to stop you from trying though – only you know your audience.

If you would like to try to challenge yourself and your riders like that, I will again direct you to the ICA website where there are various suggestions of what games you can play in your class.

Tour de France

The Tour de France provides a great opportunity every year to bring the excitement into your studio. It provides an extra subject for conversations so you can connect more with your riders.

It can provide a background for a specific technique you may want to focus on like climbing, Time Trial or Team Time Trial etc. You can work on threshold efforts, ask people to catch the TT on TV or online paying attention to the technique, level of effort, RPM etc and do an FTP test after the TT stage airs.

If you work with visuals and the technology available allows you to play a video of the stage, you are onto a winner.

I buy the *Tour de France* magazine that details every stage, describes each team and gives background to the lead rider of each of them. It also contains a big map, usually some posters of riders or vintage pictures and a pair of socks or a bandana or other trinkets. I use the profiles and adapt them to the indoor cycling format and use the items that come with the magazine as prizes in these special classes.

If you think that it would be too much of a task to create a Tour de France themed profile (especially if you want to match it with some themed music) then you should sign up to the ICA who have a vast library of Tour de France rides and playlists dating few years back that they update every year. You will get a pdf document containing the profile with cues and a matching playlist. It's a phenomenal resource.

Special rides

I have done a few of these and they have always been between 60 and 90 minutes. For that reason, we did them outside of the timetable. This means the riders have to pay to attend. Sometimes I combine these with charity collections including a donation amount in the fee for the class.

These rides are all about experience, so they are a bit different from regular classes. There is more freedom of how you ride them, music is at the very centre of it and the narrative or visualisations are the key. It's about the journey within yourself.

If you create one yourself, it is imperative to craft them carefully and have a message running throughout. Try and make them as authentic as you can, that is important in every class you teach but never more so than in a special ride like this, to make it believable. Do not just learn a bunch of empty Instagram quotes by heart and read them out. Less is more. Whether you drop a nugget of exercise science, or some fact relating to the ride you may be simulating, give people time to digest it. Ask open questions that they can answer in their own heads. And do not be afraid to keep quiet for long periods letting the music take over.

These rides, the unforgettable ones, are super hard to create. Having visuals like a projector or lights system are super cool but you can do them without these. Mixing your own music and creating a continuous playlist is invaluable.

If you have never attended one of these, I would strongly recommend attending a fitness conference or event. You have to experience a great one to grasp the idea what your benchmark is. I attended one based on Scottish Climb created by Barry Ross a Spinning MI during an event in Blackpool about four years ago and I still use some of the tracks and I still vividly remember the video and the feeling of that ride.

This year, 2019, we are celebrating 50 years since the first Moon landing and one of the ICG master instructors Ross Philipson created (and made available on the social media) a breathtaking ride called Journey to the Stars. I have seen the profile and listened to the music and I can tell you it is a masterpiece. I cannot imagine the time it must have taken for him to create this perfect playlist and can barely believe he was so generous in making it available for his fellow instructors to use. I rode it with my guys and I hope I did it justice.

To sum up, keep an eye on social media, Spotify and Soundcloud for ideas. Follow MIs and fellow instructors, attend conferences and take other people's classes. You may stumble upon a gem.

Working with a DJ

There is a chain gym in London that has live DJ classes. I am not sure how that works as I cannot imagine *not* knowing the music that will be played. I assume you would get in touch with the DJ and agree on the playlist. That said, I saw a post on Facebook once looking for a last-minute cover for one of these.

I know one MI who has taught rides with a live DJ and even though I could not attend any of these, from the riders' feedback they have been a great success and she has worked very closely with the DJ on the playlists.

Is that something you may want to look at?

I attended two special rides in the past that included live musicians. One had a live electric guitarist and the other a live percussionist. Both were crazy good, and the live music helped create a unique experience.

CHAPTER 9

Teaching Styles

There are various teaching styles that you can experience when you ride a class as a participant. Some will suit some riders, others will not. It's about individual taste, instructor's personality and riders' goals.

If you get bums on seats by following the guidelines of your certification, then keep doing what you are doing. From a point of view of a participant I will only say one thing: as long as the class is focused on the *rider* and **not** the *instructor's ego*, you are doing it right. Let me explain what I mean by that.

A few years ago, I wanted to get a gig at one of the boutique studios that had two rooms full of shiny new Matrix IC7s, state of the art lighting and sound system. And they paid way more than regular chain gyms. I knew they offered both more dance/rhythm-based classes and performance-based ones.

I was asked to come in for a chat with the manager who was also one of the main instructors. After the chat I was supposed to take part in one of his regular classes to see what was expected of me. So far so good.

The said instructor, with the impressive physique of a weightlifter, spent the last few minutes before the class flexing his muscles and just looking amazing. What he completely forgot about was asking the riders as they were filing in, whether they needed help setting up or setting up the console, whether there were any injuries etc.

We started the class and it got worse. For 45 minutes all we heard was: 'I am on 90/100/120RPM! I am on 400 watts!!! I am on 600 watts!!!". All I wanted to scream back at him was: So what mate?! Do you want me to match it? Beat it? What do you want ME to do?!?!'

We spent 45 minutes watching this guy do his own workout that we were not privy to. He finished it exhausted. Us? Not so much since we had no idea what to do and matching his power output watt for watt was simply impossible since he was a 6–2" bloke weighing probably in excess of 100kg.

I hope this illustrates my point. Your riders must feel that you are there for *them*, to facilitate *their* workout and achieve *their* goals. It is not about you showing them how fast you can pedal or how many hundreds of watts you can produce looking smug. It's about making *their* workout clear, challenging and achievable for *them*.

Prescribed Format Versus Freestyle

If you qualify as an indoor cycling instructor with any of the major training bodies like Stages, Spinning, Schwinn, ICG or YMCA you are what is known as a *freestyler*, which means you create your own profiles and playlists. You can also create a whole periodized training plan if you want (see chapter Keeping It Real).

The other way to teach is using a prescribed format. Les Mills is the leader here. When you become a LM instructor you pay a fee and you are given the choreography, script of what and when to say and the playlist. You learn it all by heart and off you go. No creative process is involved, no trawling through YouTube looking for new songs etc.

There are smaller companies who are a bit less restrictive than LM but still give you certain moves or choreography, a specific style if you will, that may be less in line with the widely accepted standards adhered to by the main providers of the international qualifications. You will however most probably need to find your own music.

Which one is better? (from instructor's point of view)

I am afraid there is no clear-cut answer. If you like the freedom of creating your own profiles and playlists, maybe using a bit more obscure music, you will feel caged by formats like LM. Personally, there is no way that I would be learning a script for my classes and say the same thing in the same place for a couple of months until the new release. And it costs a pretty penny, too. However, if you teach many other formats you will appreciate the creative part being taken off your hands leaving you to just memorise the stuff.

One of the disadvantages is that if you ever decide to go freestyle, you may feel like you regressed to the beginner level and have no idea where to start creating a class profile from scratch.

Personally, I think if you follow a prescribed format, particularly one that you just need to deliver, it stunts your growth as an instructor. But then again, you may be happy about where you are and have no plans of taking it higher.

However, when you do your own research to keep the ideas for profiles and playlists fresh, you keep the passion going. You make choices that suit your riders and your own personality and consequently when you coach, it comes across as genuine and unique to you rather than reciting a learnt formula.

Which ones do riders prefer?

LM RPM programme has a global following so clearly people do like it a lot. It will appeal to people who like predictability: you ride a new release and then you know you will ride to this for a good few weeks.

In my classes, unless we are honing a skill for a few sessions or following a training programme culminating in an FTP test, you do not know what the profile will entail until you come into the studio and I describe it to you before we start.

I know I have lost a few people because of that but I also gained numerous followers for the very same reason.

Training Versus Exercise

This is quite a touchy subject. Most of us, freelance and freestyle instructors, are exactly that: instructors. We are *not* qualified coaches, nor do we stand on average in front of a room full of professional cyclists or iron man competitors. I know some that do, and they do it in mainstream gyms having built their following and created a training specific classes, but that is not the norm. Still most of us get a great mix of ages, genders and abilities in each class we teach and your Tuesday 6pm group may have a few new riders each week, so we are constantly faced with new people that we need to accommodate.

If you teach your class in a mainstream gym and the class is marketed as a general indoor cycling class, can you run a training programme? What would that mean for people who have no interest in structured training and just come in to exercise and get a little endorphins rush?

If your studio does not want or will not market a performance class, you can still teach it provided you make it accessible to all. How?

When preparing a profile, you need to find a goal that would appeal to someone training for a competition but also be able to *sell it* to someone who never even owned a bike.

For example, you may say the following: 'Today we will work on high cadence or high RPM, if you will, which is basically fast legs. If you ride outdoors, these drills will help you get faster on the road. If you don't, you will work up a serious sweat and really challenge yourself. It will force you to work at an uncomfortable speed yet remain in control and will leave you proud of your results at the end.'

Can you see what I mean?

What Makes You Unique?

Every instructor develops their own personal style over the years. They hone their skills, pick up catch phrases and their name gets associated with certain things when mentioned by the riders in the changing rooms.

We touched on this subject earlier on. Your trademark may be music that nobody else uses, creating playlists that perfectly matches every interval. It may be that you use visualisations or your unique sense of humour. It may be the fact that each of your classes has a clear purpose that is always stated at the start and the results discussed at the end. You may be known as the one who is always there greeting everyone and setting everyone up. Or always using a cowbell …

> *Are you aware of your individual style? Do you know how riders would describe you in one sentence? Have you ever thought about how your style has evolved over the years? Or do you feel like you still need to work on it but don't know where to start?*

What helped me realise what my style was, was giving out my own feedback forms. I will talk more about them in Chapter 11.

You shape your own style by attending classes as a participant and taking part in CPD courses and Master Instructor rides. It about working out how and why something someone else does resonates with you and how you could adapt it and incorporate it into your own style.

Learn from the best

I have been extremely lucky to ride with some outstanding MIs that have been instrumental in me becoming the instructor I am today, and I will take the liberty to mention five of them here.

The main culprit responsible for getting me where I am has been **Neil Troutman** who runs Velocity Indoor Cycling certification and is a Stages Cycling MI. I came across his name on one of the FB forums and I credit him for showing me what the areas I should focus and not compromise on as an instructor are.

I admit I did not understand everything he said to me in 2012 but now, 2,500 classes later, I get it. His classes are always fun, and he always knows what to say. Not to mention the aptitude for mixing the cheesiest PPL-free music into masterpieces.

Neil was the one who introduced me to **Jennifer Sage** when she came to London to deliver a series of workshops. Most of you will be familiar with this name and the great contribution that ICA, which she established many years ago, has made to educating indoor cycling instructors globally. The vast amount of knowledge I gained from ICA articles, webinars, numerous profiles I have used over the years, cannot be overestimated and I am very proud to be able to say that I have written a few posts for them myself.

Neil was also instrumental in introducing me to Stages Cycling. During auditions to become a Stages Ambassador I met another incredible instructor. My first memory of her is when she walked into David Lloyd's Chelsea Club, fully lycra clad having just parked her bike outside and told us about getting lost on her way there. She was this super warm and smiling woman called **Janine Joseph**.

We got paired up on stage to team teach a couple of tracks and we just clicked. She is an accomplished outdoor cyclist (cycling even to nights out) and has close to 20 years' experience in teaching indoor cycling. I loved her calm demeanour, clear and understated delivery and the fact that she was so humble about it. Simon Cowell of *The X factor* would say: 'The best thing about you is that you have no idea how good you are!'

Since that momentous day I have gone to a few of Janine's classes and I learnt at least one thing from each of them that I shamelessly adapted into my own teaching style. I have since tried to deliver classes using only cool and calm Janine-tone-of-voice, but I always get too excited and end up yelling at least for a bit ... Still, my endurance rides and cues are Janine-inspired.

Then there is the Spinning MI of international fame, **Sarah Morelli**. I had the privilege of taking two rides with her at the international fitness convention in Blackpool. In a sense she's a bit like Janine. She doesn't raise her voice much or use too many words for that matter. But when she does say something, it's of substance. She is comfortable being silent for long periods and she knows the science behind indoor cycling inside out, so she can explain what she wants in very simple terms. I am a huge admirer.

Finally, there is Wattbike and Stages MI **Richard Collier**. I have taken only one class with this guy, but I watched him teach Wattbike classes for a good few months from the side lines. I used to teach at the same gym, the same day but 30 minutes later so I watched him eagerly before heading into my studio.

Richard is, as he says himself, like Marmite. You either get him or you don't. He doesn't really mince his words. If you give him your goal, he will get you to your destination, but he will be blunt about delivering a few home truths.

He was the first instructor I had seen teaching with power and really knowing his stuff. His Wattbike classes were attended by athletes as well as highly focused members of general population. He did not play any music as the bikes were in the middle of the gym and he always taught from the floor.

Watching him taught me that (1) it is possible to stay off the bike completely provided your session plan is precise and clear and (2) not everyone will like your style but if what you deliver is of value, you will build an audience if you stay true to yourself and keep getting better at what you do. Thank you, Richard.

Can you name an instrumental person or people in your career as an instructor? If you don't have anyone like that yet, go and find them. You won't regret it.

CHAPTER 10
Feedback Forms

I came across this idea a few years ago listening to a podcast with Cameron Chinatti on ICI Pro. It's a great podcast and you should check it out. Cameron is amongst other things a Master Trainer for Stages Cycling. In that episode she talked about having her own feedback forms that she would give out periodically to her riders. I really liked the idea, but I was apprehensive about it at the same time. Would people bother filling it in? Would I like what they wrote?

I decided to bite the bullet and created a form for my riders using Cameron's suggestions. You can really make this questionnaire your own and put as many or as few questions as you want. You can make them multiple choice or open ended.

I leave them all open ended because I want people to have a chance to have their say.

The things I ask about are:

- What makes me stand out from other instructors of the same format?
- Do I talk too much or too little? (yeah, right – too little!)
- What is my catchphrase? (this was the best question as the answers are so unexpected.)
- Are my instructions clear or could they be better?
- Am I motivating enough? What do I do that makes you push that extra?
- Are you bothered by me teaching off the bike?
- What about my music choices?
- Do you have any specific music suggestions?
- Would you like to see more/less of certain type of drills?

You can add as many questions as you want but bear in mind that these days people may not want to spend 15 minutes filling in this form.

I usually print a bunch of these sheets and bring them over one week a year into all my classes with a box of pens and ask people to fill them in before or after the class. People who are keen to have their input but do not have time to spare, leave me their e-mail address or take my card to contact me via social media. I then send them the same form and give them the freedom of sending their answers by any channel that is convenient for them (always give a deadline).

Then comes the fun part: crunch time! You need to be in a good mood, have some time to yourself, with possibly a glass of wine, and you start going through all these responses. It can feel a bit weird. You may feel a bit apprehensive – what if they tell me I am rubbish? Trust me, if you were really that bad, they would not bother filling those in.

I have learnt a lot over the years by analysing the feedback. It helped me to get better at my job by building on my strengths and improving the weaker areas.

I would highly recommend you going through this exercise. And keep your old forms – going through them a few years down the line is going to show you how much you have grown as an instructor.

CHAPTER 11

Keeping It Real

'Keeping it Real' is a title of an e-book written by Jennifer Sage and it's a phrase that has been adopted by the indoor cycling world. It is synonymous with keeping your indoor cycling rides as like the outdoor ones as possible, which means avoiding any contraindicated moves. These include press ups, squats, excessive or very low cadences, using weights, bars or resistance bands while on the bike.

This is always going to remain a touchy subject that will divide the indoor cycling instructors so if you are an advocate of the more 'creative' school that encourages using weights on the bike, for example, you may want skip the rest of this chapter or you risk elevating your blood pressure.

What Does it Mean to Bring Outdoors In?

Some of you will say from the start: **not everyone is a cyclist,** and it applies both to instructors and participants. There is no point in using visualisation techniques or referring to things like: 'now it should feel like you are riding to a headwind/sidewind,' or 'it's like you are drafting,' if most of your riders don't own a bike and the last time they rode one was a city hire bike with their two-year old on a tricycle next to them.

There is also a phrase widely used in the instructors' circle, namely **'if you wouldn't do it on a real bike outdoors, you shouldn't do it indoors'.** It has a point, but it has been used so much as a panacea to all kinds of suggestions of how to make a spin class 'more fun' that unless it is followed by some sound arguments based on science, it just aggravates people.

If you now expect a scientific chapter on anatomy and physiology, you will be disappointed. This book is not a serious thesis based on research and I do not hold a degree in biomechanics or sports science.

However, I am a Level 3 PT, Level 5 Sports Massage Therapist and I have a keen interest in biomechanics therefore I know that science is science and there is no need to reinvent the wheel.

When I talk about bringing the outdoors in, I mean treating a bicycle, whether stationary or an outdoor one, as a bicycle, so just sit or stand on it and pedal. It is meant to work your legs and is a great cardio fitness tool. You can build strength on a bicycle, to a certain degree, but if you want to get powerful you will have to get off it and do some serious weights work. Trying to squat on a bike while riding it is *not* the same.

And even though (since Chris Froome did it a few years ago) more riders in the Tour De France can be seen squatting low on their bikes on downhills and even pedalling in that position, they do not do it to be more powerful or work any specific muscle group but use it only on descents, trying to make themselves as small as possible while still increasing speed by pedalling. And they only pedal in that position for a few seconds.

Similarly, bending your arms while pedalling seated or standing is *not* a press up and selling it as such is misleading at least.

How do you bring the outdoors in?

Firstly, focus on pedalling, riding loads in the saddle and using the correct resistance for the task at hand.

Secondly, by using profiles that either mimic an outdoor terrain, like a steady state ride from time to time, or focusing on skills that are of value outdoors like pedalling technique, high cadence, sprinting technique etc. If you have the experience you can refer to well-known outdoor racers and races. You may want to use visuals like a video of a race or a ride (technology and licencing permitting).

There has been a trend in fitness for the last few years that reflects how we live our lives now: HIIT. High intensity. Guts out. Every class. The motto is: if it doesn't make you sick, the workout is not worth doing. Full body workout in 45 minutes every session.

In this climate it takes some courage and perseverance to build your class around staying in the saddle, getting into an uncomfortable intensity and then holding it for let's say 10 minutes. Outdoors you often face a climb that will take you 10–20 minutes to complete. This type of work forces people to focus on what their bodies are doing while giving them time to analyse its response: what do I struggle with? Why? What do I like about it? Why? It keeps them accountable for their own workout.

Doing anything for longer that 10–30 seconds at a time gives riders time to establish intensity even if they do not have a console. And if they do have one, to observe the numbers and be aware how (when they still feel the same as a minute ago) their power output is affected as the fatigue sets in. Slowing things down provides opportunities for many educational moments.

Should we not teach HIIT then? I have not said that. All types of workouts have their place and purpose. Shaking things up a bit and making your body do what it is not accustomed to is a great way of getting your riders' fitness levels up.

It's not about making our riders tired; it's about making them stronger or faster or whatever it is that they want to achieve.

> *They can get* tired *on their own. They need you to* become *fitter* in the long term.

Teaching With Power

It has been a real game changer for me, and I strongly believe this is the reason why I am still so passionate about what I do and feel like I have so much more to learn. More and more studios and gyms around the world are now using bikes with power meters or at least consoles that estimate power output. In any case your riders now can see a bunch of numbers and you need to use these to yours and riders' advantage.

The market leaders when it comes to indoor bikes using power are Wattbike (the oldest and aimed mainly at individual riders), Stages and ICG (both aimed at group ex). These three provide great training programmes for instructors that are offered on purchasing the bikes. However, some studios still choose to save money by skipping the education part which results in either the consoles not being used at all, rendering having the expensive bikes pointless, or using the information the consoles provide incorrectly by setting up unachievable targets and putting riders off using data.

One thing for sure, a lot of non-cyclist instructors and riders are intimidated by power. Instructors due to lack of knowledge, riders due to lack of understanding of benefits of using power in their regular classes.

What can you do when the studio is not offering instructor training?

My own adventure with teaching with power started when a gym I was teaching at told me they were buying IC7 bikes to replace the old bikes with no data. I got extremely excited and of my own initiative I Googled the bike's manual and read it top to bottom.

I then contacted Team ICG to see if there was any training I could take even if I had to pay for it myself. It turned out they had a lot of stuff online which was great and free of charge.

Next, I started researching training with power and made sure to attend classes where these bikes were used. It turned out to be an awful experience but at the same time invaluable as it let me suffer from the frustration the riders would, if I was teaching a class using the coach by colour system, not having a clue about the power zones. I quickly understood that I had lots to learn.

All this effort paid off when the bikes finally arrived, and I was the only one knowing how to switch the console on and what the numbers on it represented. Still, I lacked confidence in my ability and didn't have the full grasp of the concept of power, so I felt frustrated and angry. I was thinking: *'This is pointless, people* don't *care about numbers, they are not cyclists! If I have to say all these extra things about numbers and colours AND talk the old way using RPE, it's like I am talking all the time! Stupid bikes! Stupid power!'*

But I persevered and five years down the line I am one of only a few instructors using coach by colour in every single class at that gym and the only one running quarterly 20-minute FTP sessions. But it took me over a year of riding these bikes multiple times a week and learning how to link RPE with the colours, until I was able to explain in simple words to anyone who asked me: I don't ride outdoors so why should I bother with these numbers?

FTP Testing

You cannot talk about teaching with power without mentioning the FTP test – functional threshold power test. You need to know your FTP if you want to use software like Stages Flight or Coach by Colour system effectively.

There are ways of predicting the values built in some bikes, but nothing beats actual testing. You can run three, five, eight, 20 or even 60-minute tests. Each of those has its place and application. Some can be done in every class, others need more mental and physical preparation. The one-hour test is not applicable when it comes to a general population and usual class duration.

I believe testing is very important. Make sure that you have done it yourself a few times before you teach it. I will not go into details here as there are whole books about it written by specialists and there are many courses out there teaching you how to perform these. Please educate yourself. Take your teaching to the next level.

How can I learn more about teaching with power?

There are many **books** to educate yourself on using power in creating classes. Some of them are really detailed and aimed at coaches rather than group ex instructors so choosing your literature depends on what you are trying to deliver. The most digestible and easiest to read has been *'The Cyclist's Training Bible'* by Joe Friel. I have been following his blog for a while, too. If you would like a proper geek-out then get *'Training and Racing with a Power Meter'* by the two main specialists in the field Hunter Allen and Andy Coggan.

I also read **articles** posted on Wattbike, Trainer Road and Training Peaks websites. I am a member of a couple of **FB forums** for power instructors which are a real goldmine of ideas and knowledge. I follow some of the coaches and master instructors I admire on social media and ask them questions whenever I have any.

If you prefer attending a **live training session** and learn things in practice, then Stages have fantastic teaching with **power courses**. I would also recommend attending any sessions organised by Life Fitness (Team ICG). ICG have an online certification, too. Then there are the **annual fitness conferences** like IDEA in the States, FIBO in Germany and various Spinning® conferences (not all rides here are done on bikes with power so check before signing up).

Finally, if a company providing training is not offering anything soon, ask for recommendations of instructors who had qualified through them and at least try to **attend a few classes as a participant**.

Word of advice: the direction in which the industry is heading means that if you do not keep up with the technology, you will run out of teaching opportunities.

Periodisation

I learnt basics about how to periodise training during my personal training qualification course.

The concept was never mentioned in my initial indoor cycling certification which is not surprising. Designing a proper periodized plan requires a serious degree of knowledge. Do not try to run before you learn how to walk. Gain confidence in writing power-based profiles, do your research, attend training and ideally find a mentor before delving into this advanced area which is more of a coach's domain than an instructor's.

It's impossible to write a *proper* periodized programme for a random group of riders that varies every week. You can still write a general plan to practise the process but when it comes to testing the outcome at the end, it may be a bit of an anti-climax.

If, however, you have an established group or run a 6–12-week training course, then this is a perfect opportunity to apply your knowledge and test your skills at writing it. Other than that, periodise programmes are written for individual riders and are based on their specific goals and around their race calendar.

If you are interested in this topic, ICA has a few articles on it. Look up Joe Friel's Training Bible mentioned above or have a chat with someone who is an experienced coach. If you do the latter though, be prepared for discussing training software like Training Peaks. Technology is everywhere. Anyone using a periodise plan will be tracking their data and analysing their progress.

Does it mean that if you have a typical group of riders where 50 percent are regulars and the other 50 percent vary from week to week, periodisation is not an option? Maybe not in the strict terms but you can still run skill-based training programmes. For example, focus on leg speed (high cadences) for six weeks. Each week the core of the session is the same, let's say three rounds of eight minutes but the number of intervals, or their length, or the length of the recoveries, or their intensities changes each week making the subsequent sessions more demanding. Follow that by a few weeks of strength training. Finally, put all of this together and run a 20-minute FTP test.

Triathlon Training and Aero Position

First, when it comes to training for a bike leg in a triathlon, indoor cycling is a great option especially if you do it on Wattbike, IC7 (or IC8) or Stages bikes. The advantage is obviously the power meter data and the way it is gathered and presented to you. Stages bikes also have the drop bars which will enable a rider to mimic the ride on their road bike even more. IC8 also have drop bars (not many places have these bikes) and so do Wattbikes.

Therefore, creating a training programme or a profile aimed at triathletes is a great idea and may expose you to a very different audience. It will also challenge your coaching skills and will push you out of your comfort zone as an instructor.

You just need to remember that experienced outdoor riders will never be able to set their indoor bike exactly like their outdoor one. Hence the popularity of various online training platforms allowing cyclists to follow training plans, being part of an online community and making the training much less of a lonely venture yet doing all that from home using their actual bike and rollers or a turbo trainer.

Nothing will replace mileage on the actual road, getting used to side winds and climbing actual hills, yet certain skills and training are better done indoors within a controlled environment eliminating the stress of traffic or bad weather.

The bike set up

I generally allow riders who I know ride frequently outdoors and are getting ready for a competition, to set up their bike how they want it. It often means the saddle is just a bit higher than average and they may keep their handlebars lower than the saddle. However, as the main principles of bike set up apply to both indoor and outdoor bikes, I may ask them if there is any specific reason for their set up. You will be surprised how many amateurs have never heard of bike set up principles.

There are articles out there on keeping the aero position on an indoor bike – please note I am not talking about aero position on your actual road bike or tri bike when used indoors. I have also followed guidelines as mentioned by Jennifer Sage and Joe Friel.

Do you need aero position?

You do not get into that position when you ride outdoors for no reason or simply because you have the tri bars installed. You only use them to get into the most aerodynamic position on a (fairly) flat road, riding with high speed and/or when riding as a part of a 'train' trying to reap benefits of drafting. You will use that position in a time trial and team time trial.

Outdoor riders do not use it when climbing or riding out of the saddle which for whatever reason seems to be the case with indoor riders. To be honest, as much as I love IC7 bikes, if I could chop off the 'tri bars' on them, I would … Using these impedes riders' breathing and encourages them to grip those bars tightly hence putting pressure on the wrists. Plus, you can hardly argue that you need to tuck in against the wind in an indoor cycling studio! (Unless you own a Shimano headwind machine, that is – how cool are those?!) And what is it with people squeezing those bars for dear life until their knuckles turn white?

What is more, sitting in a tucked in position requires certain back flexibility hence I would never ask my group to ride that way.

The thing I struggle with the most is understanding when people whose set up is awful (handlebars so high that they are practically sitting upright) use the tri bars which means that their elbows are on the bars. It's extremely uncomfortable so why do it? The reason must be the subconscious urge to cheat: if your handlebars are too high and you lean on them, you take pressure off your legs making it feel easier to turn the legs around faster. But then your upper body gets tense and tired. As a result, you end up with riders going at high RPM and insufficient resistance who by the end of the class feel their arms, wrists and shoulders hurt, and which they interpret as upper body part of the workout.

Should you, or shouldn't you?

There is a great article on bicycling.com titled *'How Aero is Too Aero?'* It talks about how the level of your torso angle influences your power output. Granted, it is more of importance to highly trained athletes, but the principles remain the same.

If that is too much of a scientific approach to the topic, then read the ICA article *'Another Reason NOT to Ride Aero in a Spinning Class'.* It does a great job of putting it in layman terms. To paraphrase it, you squash your insides including the diaphragm which is crucial to maintaining the correct breathing on a bike. Also as the bike underneath you does not bend or move like an outdoor bike does, there are various sheering forces that are being transferred to your elbows, shoulders, and lumbar spine disks which can lead to injuries or health issues long term: elbows, shoulder pain, lower back pain.

To summarise, serious outdoor cyclists and triathletes used to riding aero outside, will often default to this position in the warm up and in endurance rides. However, many soon realise they cannot get the same set up and feeling as on their own actual road bike (completely different frame dimensions) and will sit with their hands wide. I let them be. We are group ex instructors not qualified coaches or bike fitters so we can only give advice based on what we learn from experts and our own research. If someone is trying to create a third leg (using their arms and the handlebars) to offload their existing two, I correct them. Ultimately, if someone then decides to ignore your advice it is their choice.

When People Do Contraindicated Stuff.

You know by now that I am one of those instructors whose classes are ridden mainly in the saddle. Other than that, we are out of the saddle. That's it. No upper body choreography. I don't use the word 'choreography' when I refer to cycling classes at all. We do not ride at excessively high or low cadence. All my regular riders know it and if anyone asks around the gym about my classes, people will tell them that it is all just cycling. I have science to back it up – take it or leave it.

When someone comes to my regular class, they will not get an opportunity to do any contraindicated moves *unless* they choose to go rogue and start doing something of their own volition. When I see that, I will correct it by bringing it to their attention. If it continues, I will say that we do not do it in this class and should the person performing the move wish to discuss the reasoning behind it, they are more than welcome to approach me after the class. If that does not make them stop, I will approach them and firmly request for them to stop and follow my advice.

If however they don't, I will make a point of bringing it up in a cool down and say to the whole group that if my style of teaching is not what suits them, they are free to choose other instructors but politely ask them not to come again unless they agree to stop doing whatever that was that goes against my training. I will take my time to explain the science behind my reasoning.

Harsh? Maybe, but I know what I ask of my riders and why. I also know why I don't ask them to do certain moves. Don't get me wrong, you get loads of freedom in my classes: you can sit the whole session, you can stand up when I cue it or when your bum needs a break. You can choose to do every second interval if you feel you need more recovery. You can ride a zone lower in intensity if you're not up to it or are riding a recovery ride. You can go up a zone if I know this is what your training plan dictates. When I ask for a 'fast flat' I say it should be RPM that feels fast to *you* so it will be between 80–110RPM depending on your fitness and goals. That's enough freedom, isn't it?

But there is a reason I am on the other side of the room and that is my qualification backed up by my insurance and code of ethics. If what you are trying to do goes against these rules, even if other instructors or studios do it, I will not have it in my class.

What if I only cover a one-off class?

Sometimes you must pick your battles. You may disagree with a style but don't make it personal towards an instructor so I will not be saying: 'Your regular teacher Jane is a bad instructor and you should stop going to her classes!' If I get a sense (or know from my research) that contraindicated moves are a norm in that class, I am prepared to see them and will still ask people not to do them but I choose not to get overly stressed about that or get too preachy. I will encourage people to try it my way but at the end of the day I am only there for that one hour and may never see these people again.

I have not always been like that. Remember the story from the Confessions chapter? I once agreed to cover for an instructor who was big on contraindicated moves, for two weeks. I spent the whole 45 minutes repeating: 'Don't do this! Don't do that! That is not the right way!', making it the most negative class I have ever delivered, and the participants ever ridden. At the end I was mentally exhausted, and people were miserable having been constantly berated. The following week when I came back, a lady who had been there the previous week walked in, saw me and said: 'Oh, no! I can't do that!' and she left. That was my lesson.

If I agree to cover a class that is all about the upper body, I tell the riders at the start that there will be no upper body moves in this class and as it is one off, they should really give it a try. Worst case scenario and they don't like it as much as their regular class, it is only this once then the normal order resumes. I will not actually insert a few press ups or dips or anything like that. I cannot do it. I do not believe that type of a cycling workout to be safe and efficient, so I stick to what I know. Take it or leave it. My inability to compromise in this respect cost me a few potential permanent and well-paid classes but I couldn't agree to sell out.

Some of you may be getting quite upset at this point as using weights and upper body moves is indeed the style you teach and have been successful in building a great following. There is a place on the market for everyone. I know why this way of riding does not sit well with me so we can all agree to disagree and move on.

Let's bust some myths

Riding a bike uses a whole body. Correct but mainly legs. The rest is used to keep you seated or standing. You need your hands and arms to hold on to the bike, but they are not getting a 'workout' per se.

There are places offering indoor cycling classes that target the whole body making it a full body workout (using weights, resistance bands or bars).

Let me say it one more time: you *do* activate most of your body when riding a bike (especially outdoors when balancing is necessary). However, unless part of your session involves getting off your indoor bike and lifting it above your head or lying on the floor chest pressing it, it will never be a full body workout, as it will not help you build strong triceps, biceps or pectoral muscles.

I actually get quite angry when I see some places advertise on social media using women fitness models with ripped abs or guys with massive biceps and traps making you believe that they look the way they do because they lift 0.5 lbs weights on a bike five times a week for 10 minutes. I applaud these models for keeping their physiques so impressive as it requires a great effort and discipline when it comes to working out and even more, nutrition. Teaching indoor cycling classes is *helping* them to keep in shape but if they were doing *only* that, the way they do it, they would look different. No doubt about it.

Riding a bike, you need to consciously engage your core by bracing it

I am a rider and an instructor. I have also taken many Pilates classes. Yet when it comes to riding a bike, 'bracing my core' makes no sense. As my colleague Stevie Barr who is a biomechanics coach would say, the core is able to take care of itself. Since you are not falling off the bike the core *is* engaged. It would be more beneficial to remind people to breathe deep using their diaphragm and letting their belly hang out.

Many times, I have seen women riders in my classes wearing crop tops, sporting great physiques, doing that bracing thing which makes them tense up their upper body, stick their butts out and generally look very stiff. (I mention their dress code as it makes it easier to see than if they were wearing a loose T-shirt).

If your knee jerk reaction to this example is to respond that this is not what you mean when you ask your riders to brace their core, could you explain specifically what it is that you do mean? Do you explain it clearly every time you cue it? Before I did my first Pilates class, I had never heard about bracing your core and would have no idea at all about what it implied if asked to do that in a cycling class.

In Pilates they explain it as drawing navel to your spine, tightening everything, while still breathing normally. If I do *that* in a cycling class, I won't be able to breathe as deep as I need for a cardio workout, in an endurance ride or worse even a sprint effort.

So, if you use this cue, how do you explain it? Do *you* know what you mean and what you want the riders to do exactly or do you think you have to say it because other instructors do?

You need a strong core to be a strong cyclist

Damn right you do but you will need to strengthen it off the bike. Yoga, Pilates, body balance etc. Remember that 'core' is not only abs. You need your back to be strong and flexible to comfortably lean forwards from your hips.

CHAPTER 12
Intensity

This chapter is about what makes bread and butter of our work. How hard do we make our classes and more importantly, how do we convey the intensity we want the riders to achieve? Is it good to be known as the instructor who makes riders feel physically sick at the end of each class? This will inadvertently lead to the subject of recovery as there can be no conversation about one without the other.

How to Describe Intensity Zones

Some of you who are not lucky enough to teach on bikes with consoles, let alone coach by colour or Stages Flight or Intelligent Cycling systems, may be tempted to skip this part thinking that with no data to keep track on, there are no intensity zones to refer to. That assumption would be incorrect.

If you work with no power meters or consoles at all and all you have is the RPE scale, your job is harder, but you still should know intensity zones. These are basically the same as power zones but the vocabulary you would be using do describe them is different. When you work with power and FTP you may cue: 'Zone 3', 'tempo ride', 'VO2max intervals' or 'over 130% FTP'. Without power data you rely solely on the RPE scale – rate of perceived exertion.

The most common one is 1–10. Some use 1–5 version others prefer 1–20. I always found the 1–20 too wide. The shortest 1–5 version, even though it would correspond to the basic five power zones, was never my favourite but use whatever you are most comfortable with and whatever your riders are used to.

The main disadvantage of RPE is that it is totally subjective. It relies on people paying close attention to their body's response to the exercise. Some riders are not used to it and find it hard to gauge their effort even on the scale 1–10. Use any tools at your disposal to help them.

The main way to establish where they are on the scale is a talk test. How do you perform a talk test on 40 riders? Ask them an open question that they should answer loud enough so they can hear it under their breath. Can they get a full sentence out? Great, they are still between easy and moderate effort level. If they can only utter a few words before they need to breathe, we are around hard work level. If only one word comes out or all they can do is grunt and give you evils, we are up there 9–10RPE. Different responses, different intensities.

I would not leave it all to the talk test though. Talk about how the legs are feeling – smooth and steady stroke or more engagement from the hamstrings? Can they hear their breathing? Is their mouth slightly open or is it hanging open as they try to get as much oxygen in as possible?

I must say that even though I work with power in 99% of my classes and coach by colour system in 90% of my classes, I still use RPE in all of them. You cannot really teach using power zones unless you understand fully what each zone feels like, how long it is sustainable for and where each of them falls on the 1–10 scale.

How to make RPE work

- Be consistent.
- Be clear.
- Be descriptive.

My advice is to make sure that whatever RPE you are used to using, make sure you are consistent and very clear as per what each number stands for. When I take a class as a participant and all I hear is: 'Give me 7!' I still don't know what that means unless it's followed by a context or if a handout explaining each number is available for me to refer to.

Some instructors believe it's enough to say: 'We start from 5. Then we will go up from here'. I have seen instructors asking people to max the resistance up to the point their legs stop and say: 'This is 10. Now take it down and find 5'. With all due respect this is all meaningless and I guarantee you everyone in that room is on a different intensity level and is unable to describe to you where on the scale of 1–10 they are.

To use any RPE efficiently you must be clear about what is 1 and what is 10. My favourite phrase is: '*1 – you are on a sofa eating chips. 10 – you are dead.*'

I would recommend printing the RPE you want to use and make sure you can describe in a maximum of two sentences what each number should feel like. You can put those notes next to the numbers and make sure you say them enough times, so they come out in your sleep. Again: be consistent! If your six today means that I can: 'hold a conversation, but I am getting really warm,' and tomorrow it's, 'hard work,' then it's not helpful.

How do you find the right description? You can Google what other people use but there is no substitute for experiencing each zone. I really got well versed in describing intensity only after I started riding with power. If you have a chance to take a few classes focused around power and using power zones with qualified and experienced instructors, and ideally do an FTP test (of any length), you will gain the best insight into what each zone feels like.

Make sure you can describe each intensity in terms of:

- RPE scale.
- Breathing (deep and long breaths/open mouth, slightly laboured/breathing like a train/gasping for breath).
- Talk test (you can hold a full conversation/you can talk but breathing is changing/you can say an incomplete sentence/you can say two to three words/you can only grunt/you can only give me the finger without letting go of the handlebars).
- What do the legs feel like? (legs are fine it's more of a change in breathing/flat road/you are struggling to keep the RPM at 64–66/feel pressure under your feet/you can feel your hamstrings working/legs are burning and you can't wait for this to end).
- Corresponding colour used by your console or PIQ, of applicable percentage of the FTP.
- Recovery (you get 2/3/6/10 minutes and you should need them to completely recover/you get 30 seconds and it shouldn't feel like a complete recovery).

You need to know these inside out. For each zone or intensity level, if you will. If you ride short intervals of let's say 15–30 sec, you may be better off describing the intensity zones you will be moving between *before* you start the first interval or even the class. When you ride long ones, you can use different references to keep riders engaged and have something useful to say. For example:

We will go 30 seconds on, 30 seconds off. On is Zone 4, yellow, hard work. FTP% 95–100%. Legs quite heavy, but you are not gasping for breath, just starting to hear it. Off is Zone 2, recovery zone, blue. Feels great but it is not a complete break. Legs feel light, breathing calms down. FTP% 56–75%.

Of course, the reference to percentage of FTP and colours are used when applicable, but knowing them back to front, means you will be able to teach on any bike to any group. I now refer to percentage FTP automatically – even if I teach without consoles! It's just my second nature.

If you are thinking that this is a whole lotta talking – you don't need to say all these things at once. If your interval is more than 2-3 minutes, use a different phrase every 30 seconds or a minute. Use body language, exaggerated facial expressions, etc.

Mastering this knowledge means you remain consistent, and your clear message gets to all the riders: those who use and love numbers and those who prefer descriptions.

It is also extremely useful when you teach with power and colour zones, but you get new riders who have not done their FTP test and simply used an estimation of their threshold. It is a common occurrence that the prediction is way off and consequently their console or gauge on the screen is permanently in red/purple zone (implying they are in Zone 7 and should be approaching clinical death) while they really are in Zone 3. Or their face is purple, and they are gasping for breath while the data claims that they are still in recovery zone.

When teaching with colours I always give the caveat that first timers should match my guidelines on RPM, then my description of what I want them to feel like by adding or taking off resistance and *then* check what colour it gives them compared to what colour the feeling *should* correspond with. If the feeling is right but the colour is off, go with the feeling. Then at the end of the class they can approach me and discuss which way the number was off, and I can advise them on what to change it to next time.

You will hear me say the following: 'the colours on your screen are extremely useful and meaningful, provided that the right data has been entered under the threshold. If it's not and your console is red (IC7) or the gauge on the big screen is purple (Stages) for 45 minutes, that doesn't mean you should be fast tracked for the next Olympics but simply that the numbers entered into the system were too low.

Can I Teach a Whole Class at the Same Intensity?

This is a question I have seen online, and it resonated with me for two reasons. Firstly, I thought that it should be obvious but that was a bit presumptuous. Secondly, it's not that common in the era of instant gratification and HIIT workouts to do that.

Let's tackle the issue then. Is it possible to keep the same intensity throughout the 45- or 60-minute class? It is but you need to have the knowledge of intensity or power zones to know which are sustainable for the given time.

Zones 1 to 3, so all the way to around 90% of the FTP (threshold), are great for endurance rides and can be sustained for up to a few hours. I do not know anyone who would like to ride for an hour or more in Zone 1 (below 55% FTP) simply because it is not challenging and holding it for that long would make it boring.

Zone 2 which is the recovery zone is good for just that – long recovery rides.

Zone 3 spans from 76–90% FTP and I call it the sweaty zone. This is where your breathing gets deep, after five minutes or so the mouth starts to open as you are expelling the excess CO_2. This is an aerobic zone, so you rely on oxygen as your fuel. Your legs feel fine for a long time. You can still hold a conversation, but your body temperature rises steadily and as a result you sweat a lot. In my experience you need to hold this zone for 10-minutes or more to fully appreciate it. And you feel the effect of it in your legs when you *get off* the bike.

Zone 4 is the threshold zone ranging from 91–105% FTP. Your strong and experienced riders may be able to hold it for up to an hour. But to an average population it will not be achievable.

Zones 5–7 are sustainable in minutes or barely seconds, so they are out of the question in this scenario.

I love using long intervals in Zones 3 and 4 in my classes. These rides bring focus, allow riders to get a proper feel of each intensity and appreciate that they do not need to sprint to get a great workout. This type of a ride also makes a difference from the constant, 'Go! Go! Go!' type of a class which may be challenging.

It is definitely a challenge for the instructors as coaching long intervals in the same intensity requires skill, thought and imagination. As an instructor you need to hold your nerve and not be tempted to up the intensity to break the monotony. It is also the time to learn to be silent. You don't want to be talking throughout a 10- or 20-minute interval. Allow people to get in their zone. Set them free but keep an eye on them. Perfect opportunity for walking around and one to one coaching. With experienced riders and in coach by colour classes I don't even mind if they listen to their own music.

We Don't Need No Stinking Recoveries!

When referring to intensity, recovery is the key term. Recovery does not have to be complete it may be just backing off slightly. It will all depend on which intensity zone you are working in and how long for.

As a qualified instructor you should know work to rest ratios. I know it is brought up during teaching with power courses but I believe that if your cueing is on point and you are able to really guide your riders to the intensity you want them at even without power meters, then you should apply the official guidelines on recovery.

Anytime I hear or see a post online from an instructor who says that their groups don't like recoveries and they don't need them, I really want to scream. That means that either they ride at too low intensities or the instructor's cueing is unclear or what they are asked to do is indeed so easy they really do not need recoveries.

I admit it's much easier to teach people the value of recoveries when you teach with power meters. If you ask for a series of 10 intervals at VO2 max and ask the riders to achieve the same power output in each and every single one, they see very clearly when that power starts dropping or nosediving. When you only work with RPE this is not as obvious as it still *feels* like you are working just as hard.

Does it mean there is nothing you can do when you ride old school bikes? Not at all. I just take extra time to really spell out the level of effort I need, especially in terms of breathing. In particular, when talking about power/intensity zones 5–7, I will mute the music after the third or fourth interval and say: 'I need to hear your breathing. By now you can hear it loud and clear. By next round you will hear the person next to you. Sometimes in maximal efforts I will mute the music at the end of the 10–15 sec interval and say: "Can you hear it? Can you feel it now? It was OK while you were doing it, right?" Well, it hurt in the thighs, true, but now the HR is over the roof, the sweats are coming, and the breathing is all over the shop, isn't it? It is not? When are you planning to start sprinting then?'

On longer intervals of 3–10-minutes at threshold I choose songs where the beat drops in the middle and the music goes quiet. I then say: 'can you hear your body? This is the sound of hard work. Do not hold it in, if you want to say something or even swear a little, if it helps you to maintain this effort, then do it. Be proud of how hard this is and that you are sticking with this discomfort and not giving up. Can you hear the person next to you? If your body is totally silent and your mouth shut, and you are honest with yourself, is this really hard work? Is this what you came here to do?'

Then the recovery comes and it's more or less the same message I give my riders: I only give you the recovery you need to achieve the goal of this ride. I would not give you five-minutes recovery if you only needed 60 seconds so if you only do need 60 seconds, make sure you work harder in round two. In the meantime, if you are ready, increase intensity and go just hard enough so you don't feel like you are wasting your time or getting bored. Then make sure you step on it in the next interval. Don't just get tired. Be smart in your workout and make sure you see improvements long term. For that you need recovery.

What do you do to keep people engaged during recoveries?

If they worked as hard as you wanted them to, they don't need to be entertained during an adequate recovery as they will use it fully to get their breath back and be ready for what is coming next.

If the recovery track is long, 5–10-minutes, you can summarise what was done and what is coming. I use open questions that I leave for each rider to answer in their heads: 'what was the hardest part of that last interval? Was it holding the high RPM or the resistance? Were the legs fine but breathing was the problem, or the other way around? Could you hold this intensity for another 10s/30s/60 seconds? We are now halfway through the recovery – is your HR back to normal? Are you able to hold a conversation? What does that mean since you have another x minutes available?'

I also use that time to refill people's water bottles, walk around and see if anyone needs any help or clarification on anything. Let the riders chat and compare notes if they want to.

What if the planned recovery seems too short or too long?

If I use a new profile or teach without data or maybe the air conditioning is not working and with the full studio the room temperature and humidity reach unsafe levels I may either add to the recovery or shorten it slightly. I simply watch people's faces and bodies and make the assessment. If I think the recovery is too long as I can see people getting restless and distracted, I first reassess my cueing of the intensity. It only happens when I teach one-off classes without any data and people are not used to tuning in with their bodies' responses.

Don't Touch My (Resistance) Knob!

What I am talking about here is an instructor walking up to a rider and turning their resistance up for them if they feel the rider is not working within the right intensity zone.

I need to tread carefully here as I have been guilty of a gross misconduct in this area once. It was a few years back and I still remember it like it was yesterday. I had a new rider in who was sitting there smiling and bouncing happily in the saddle, completely ignoring my cues both verbal and visual. I went up to her a couple of times trying to indicate with my whole body and clapping to the beat I wanted her to hold and she would still not do anything. Finally, I said to her off the mic: 'if you want to get any workout you really need to add some resistance'. To which she responded with a smile: It doesn't go any further. And that's where I went in and out of frustration turned it up around two turns (old bikes). It did slow her legs down to where she was supposed to be, but it came as a shock to her and she stopped smiling. I went back to my bike petrified and feeling rotten. I promised myself I would go up to her and apologise at the end of the class. Unfortunately, she left when we started stretching and she never came back …

As a rule, you should never change people's resistance. Especially if you do not pay attention to their body's responses but simply *think* they should be on a certain level of resistance. I have seen instructors not giving an intensity or RPE just giving a random gear level and then walking around making sure people were on it. Horror!

What I do resort to sometimes is if I have a beginner rider who really struggles and when they take their eyes off the console to look at the resistance knob to increase it their RPM drops, their posture changes etc. Then it takes them 10–20 seconds to get back to the previous RPM by which point I may cue to bring the resistance down again. Upon recognising it, I approach them and say: 'Keep doing what you are doing, your RPM is on point. But looking at your body I can see that you are still in Zone 2 and we need to head into Zone 3 now so a bit harder. I am going to increase your resistance by 1%. Then you will decide if you think we can add another 1% so nothing drastic, OK?' I will then leave them to continue and come back to them again when I see the body's response to the intensity change and make sure I say: Well done. You see, you are stronger than you give yourself credit for.

The other day I was discussing it with a colleague who said she understood my reasoning behind it, she knows I would not whack the resistance up by a massive margin and I always tell people what I am going to do but it may be better to ask: 'May I increase your resistance by 1%?' so they feel they have the power to say no. A very slight difference but less imposing on the rider's personal space.

Chapter 13
Using Notes

Schoolteachers need to have a written lesson plan for each class they teach, at least at the beginning. With experience they may not have detailed notes for every single class, but they are following a curriculum with clear goals that will culminate in some form of assessment for their students to see what they learnt.

When you are a freelance group exercise instructor, unless you are teaching under a Les Mills licence, you do not get a lesson plan nor are you required to have one to prove to anyone that you have thought through what you are going to do with your riders for the next hour. It's *expected* that your class will have an intro, a warm up, main part and a cool down but unless you happen to work for a gym that does occasional audits (where a studio manager sits in on your class filling in a form and then asking you to sign it and discuss the feedback), nobody will ever know whether you wing it or not. Isn't that just crazy?

We are responsible for groups of people day in day out, some of us see in excess of 250 people a week, all expecting that the instructor they are looking at really knows what they are doing. That whatever they are asked to do or not to do is safe, has a point and will help them achieve their goals, whatever they may be.

What about the notes then? Should you use them?
Are they good or bad? How long should you use them for? What format? Should you study them at home or on the way to your class but never look at them while teaching?

Firstly, understand there is nothing wrong with using notes. If they help you deliver a top class, then use them.

When I first started teaching, even though I was creating typically music-driven classes (verse one thing, chorus another), I used to create a playlist on my iPad, then take a screen shot of it, print it out and add any notes. Finally, I would put that page in a clear plastic sleeve and have it in front of me at least the first few times I would use the playlist.

I know that Spinning® programme has a set of symbols that instructors use when creating profiles to minimise the amount of writing. It means your class plan looks like a code sheet for the uninitiated but can be easily borrowed by another instructor who knows the key.

I have seen various ideas used by instructors – neat general cue cards and very detailed notebooks with the class written out to the second. I say, use whatever works for you.

These days I use my iPhone for everything. I create my profiles or use ones created using colour zones on Stages Flight, ICG Training and Intelligent Cycling. These give you an instant visual overview of the ride.

If I see a profile on ICA or even Sufferfest App that I like, I adapt it using one of these platforms or just using the Notes app on my phone. Oftentimes when I see someone else's detailed notes, I cannot understand the profile well. I have to write it up my way first, to understand the structure clearly.

I also tend to write an e-mail to myself attaching a screenshot of the notes and of the accompanying colour profile. This way if my phone fails, I always have them in my inbox.

When I teach a class using Stages Flight, the riders and I can all see the profile, so no notes are necessary. Wouldn't it be great if that was a standard?

Once I have taught a profile a few times, I may create a short version of the notes simply stating the purpose, focus and the times of the intervals, RBI and intensities.

Should you keep the notes secret in class or use them at all?

Every time someone asks any notes related question on the online forums it divides the community into two camps: 'I NEVER use notes! It's UNPROFESSIONAL!' And 'ALWAYS! NOT HAVING notes is so unprofessional!'

I think the key is preparing your ride in advance. Knowing your whys and whens. Being able to say in a sentence or two what the class is about. Asking for things that are realistically achievable. If you can do it without notes – great! If you need notes – do it. I have never ever had anyone approach me to criticise my use of notes. I have however had a few comments on how riders appreciated it when a class was well thought out.

Another thing, over the years I have accumulated a vast library of playlists. As not all of them are done using the visual platforms, I catch myself going into an old one and trying to work out what the hell I was trying to achieve there. I then look for the notes that went with it. Check out Chapter 8 on Music to get advice on hiding your notes in the title of the song or the profile.

How do you display your notes?

I use my phone that I put on the handlebars. I tried one of those holders that you attach to the handlebars but as I use the phone as a timer, when your phone is suspended like that sometimes it does not react to swiping. The downside of having the phone lying directly under your face is that the dripping sweat makes the screen switch sometimes or makes it stop reacting altogether. Thankfully I ride with consoles 99% of the time so I can use the timer on the console and keep the phone to the side just to glance at the structure or a cue list.

Keiser bikes have got a great tablet size holder on the bars which I love. I love Stages bike but the only place to put your phone on is either inside the low bottle holder which renders it invisible, or on top of the actual console which renders the console invisible. It is not an issue if you have the Flight system but if you are using the app, it can get annoying so please Stages, think about it when making any future improvements!

To sum up, notes are extremely useful. They allow you to visually assess the profile before you ride it. Creating a profile on paper or software and then riding it also helps you understand that something that looks good in theory may not work in practice.

How detailed your notes are depend on you. One thing to avoid or wean yourself off doing as you gain experience, is to rely on extremely detailed notes accounting for every second of the class. Memory joggers are great, but you don't want to sound like you are reading from a script and not looking at your riders once, for fear of losing your place.

Do not let anyone bully you into thinking you must or mustn't have notes or you are a bad instructor!

Using notes to expand your vocabulary

This is what I use notes a lot for. This issue is raised by many instructors who feel like they say the same thing over and over. To remedy it, write down any quotes of phrases you think would fit in to your class and then have them in front of you when you teach. When you find a suitable moment, use them. Keep the cheat sheet until your vocabulary expands and you no longer need the prompts. ICA has a great list of 100 cues that you can get from their website.

When you forget your notes

It can be detrimental to teaching your class if you are riding a profile for the first time. This has never happened to me as I put my notes in the playlist's title but if you forget your cheat sheet you may need to use a different profile or use the same playlist but work out what you can do with it to make it work even if it is very different from the original intention.

That is why it's important not to rely solely on the notes. Use them as a crutch or a safety net but make sure you know what you are going to do without them. Use them to make things run super smooth.

CHAPTER 14

Motivating the Riders

We can look at motivation from two angles: how to motivate your riders and how to stay motivated as an instructor.

Let's talk about motivating the riders first. The first thing that springs to mind immediately is **music**.

We are all DJs in this business. To keep sane, we need to remember that we will never please everyone. A playlist that rocks one studio may fall flat in another, even though the average age of the riders is the same. I would say that if the instructor enjoys their own music it comes across. More importantly, if the music fulfils its purpose in your class, the mission is accomplished. Go back to Chapter 8 to read more about music.

The next thing crucial in motivating the group in front of you, is **your personality**. Clients will follow an instructor even if their classes are not the most effective, purely because of who they are as a person. If they are fun, full of energy and develop a connection with the participants, they can motivate them to do anything.

As an instructor, your **energy levels** must be top in every class. You need to leave your private issues outside to make it all about the clients for the duration of the session. You don't have to be the cheering and whooping type of instructor. Your strength may be in being focused, levelled and methodical about delivering your programme. Whatever makes you, you – bring it on (see Chapter 10).

Finally, what really motivates many riders (not all) are **results**. If you give them a chance to test their fitness level, give them an opportunity to work on their skills, then retest and see an improvement, you will have soaring levels of motivation across the board.

When you're teaching a very small group and their motivation is zero.

The most challenging situation you can come across is a small group of riders, maybe in a one-off cover class, whose motivation is rock bottom. Basically, trying to energise them is like bleeding a stone. They refuse eye contact and look like they'd rather be anywhere else. They may be really deflated by you being there instead of their regular instructor. Or if you are a high energy level person and their regular instructor is not, they are used to a flatline type of coaching and are not used to seeing or showing any type of enthusiasm.

I remember teaching a class once at 9am, which was my second class of the day, and I had a fasting ultrasound booked for 2pm so I could not eat or drink *anything* apart from water. I warned the group (who didn't know me) before we started that I was already feeling a bit spaced out so would be taking it easy. I was off the bike for the most of that class yet at the end two people approached me and said: 'This was you on low energy levels?! I am not that awake after a double espresso!'

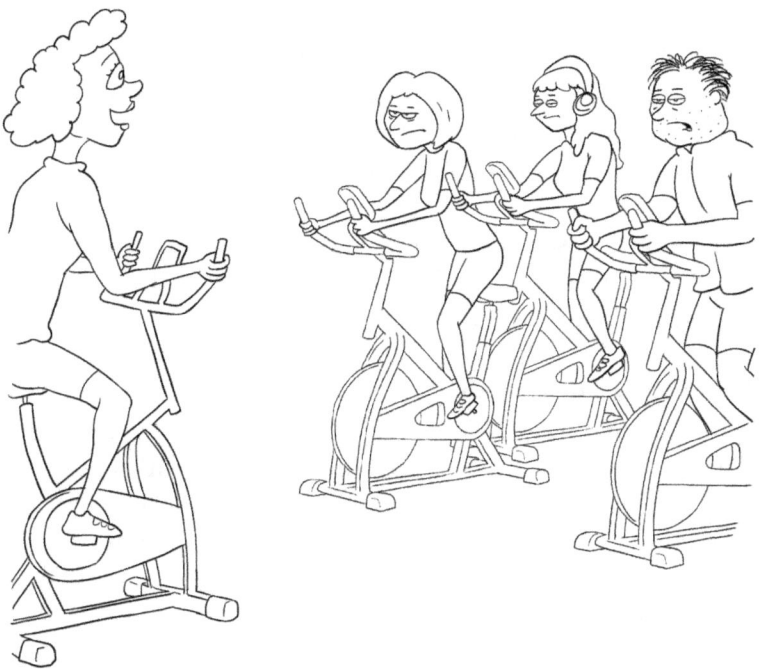

Going back to a group of 'zombie' riders. If there are a few of those among the group, it is not a problem but sometimes you only get a small group of 4–6 riders and it's made up fully of 'zombies'. I mean: no interest, zero connection, no willingness to put up any resistance on their bikes, 15-minutes in and their breathing still has not changed and most of all they look bored out of their brains. I swear, these classes are the most exhausting for me as an instructor. I try every technique I have in my toolbox to get a spark out of these people as I don't have it in me to just give up on them and simply make it my own workout session by ignoring them back. Still, you can only do so much. When the ordeal is over, thank the universe this is just a one-off and if possible, have a nap.

What if it's not a one-off and it is a new permanent class you have accepted? Good luck!

I didn't mean it. I mean I did. A group like that may take months to bring to life. First thing is to understand what made them 'die inside' and what they would like to do. I swear to God it may feel like working in a quarry. There should be a financial bonus for turning a group like that around.

Sometimes though it may be better for everyone if you move on. I have had a couple of permanent classes in the past where after a few months of hard graft and exasperation (only on my behalf) I realised that I wasn't suited to that demographics. I was getting frustrated and realised I was not looking forward to teaching there. They were all about wearing designer gear and loads of make-up and although they were really focused, their focus was on keeping the make-up and hairstyle intact for 45-minutes.

Instructor's motivation

Let me put this out there first – for 99% of us it is *not* the money as we do not get paid enough. It's a fact! In the UK the market rate paid per 45-minute class across gyms and studios has remained unchanged for about 20 years. There are places paying much more but they require you to incorporate contraindicated movements and since I will not compromise on that, I get paid the minimum.

To tie back motivation to the point above about teaching a

non-responsive class, I think riders do not realise how much the instructor feeds off the energy given off by the group in front of them. When I read interviews with singers who talk about the thrill of performing and interacting with a crowd, the energy high and the come down after they get off the stage, I can relate to it. And it doesn't have to be an international showcase. I get the feeling every time I get in front of the group. And when the music, the profile, the energy levels and the interaction all come together, you leave the studio floating on cloud nine. If the riders give you nothing, it all just feels flat.

When numbers are low

First, is it a new development or have you taken over a poorly attended slot? If the class used to be busy and suddenly the numbers have dropped the reasons may be anything: time of the year, school holidays, new gym or a new studio opening close by and giving out free passes, the standard of the facility declining (cleanliness, sauna closed, air conditioning not working, etc.). Talk to the riders and talk to other instructors – is this a trend or is it just your slot? Talk to the management. Maybe it's time to step up promotion or announce a new initiative? Check Chapter 9 for special class ideas. But if you work out (or suspect) that it may be that you are not a good fit for the place, it may be better to move on.

Instructor's block

We have all heard about writer's block (thankfully I have not experienced this when writing this book) but what about instructor's block? It's a term I see quite often on the forums.

I think to prevent this from happening you need to **continue your education** and always expand your professional skills. Learning about teaching with power and creating profiles based on intensity rather than music can be game changers. I am not trying to bring down instructors who start creating their rides from music as I used to do that, too but there is a limit to it. Even if you have one thousand songs in your library, you can only do as much using verse/chorus changes. Furthermore, one class does not lead to the next as is just a stand-alone workout. This limits you. If you have a profile in mind which focuses on a specific skill, then you can play with it by increasing its intensity each week. And no, you do not need power meters to be able to do it. You can simply shorten the recovery tracks and squeeze in another work track. (See the chapter on Intensity)

Another way of **keeping things fresh** is **attending classes** as a participant and seeing how others teach.

If you need music inspiration, the **online FB forums** are great for that. You can also follow other instructors on Spotify.

For more profile ideas go to Chapter 7.

If your block is a result of you teaching multiple classes every day and simply feeling burnt out, **stepping away** for a while may be what is needed. If you can, give up a few classes at least temporarily so you get excited to teach again rather than deflated.

How to stay passionate about teaching?

As with any area of your life, if you think you have learnt everything there is to learn about a subject, you will get bored sooner or later. However, **you cannot have too much education**. Whether it's **reading up on the latest research, attending events and seminars, reading books** or using the goldmine of easily accessible knowledge that is the **ICA website**, you can always learn more and become better at what you do.

The fitness industry is very dynamic and as such it keeps evolving. New research studies are being conducted all the time and innovative fitness concepts keep popping up even within the indoor cycling industry itself. Not everything that is new is worth taking on board but to make a conscious decision of what is viable and can bring positive results for your clients, you must have a sound knowledge of what it is that you teach.

Unfortunately, to become an indoor cycling instructor (in the UK) it is enough to have level 2 gym instructors qualification plus an indoor cycling training module, which can be as short as a half day training and there is no prerequisite to having taken indoor cycling classes prior to the training. You just tick 'yes' box next to 'Have you been taking regular cycling classes?'

Many instructors complete that basic training, and this is where they stay as far as their education in the field goes. I know some who did their course 10 years ago and have never updated their knowledge as it is not required and they live by the statement: 'It's riding a bike, what new can I learn?' A friend of mine who teaches Pilates said to me once that she could not teach indoor cycling as there is nothing to teach. Isn't there?

When I qualified over eight years ago, even though it was on Keiser bikes with consoles, the concept of power training was not even mentioned. Three years later most of London gyms got Matrix IC7s or Stages bikes and ©Stages Flight software, studios with Schwinn and Keiser bikes use various PIQ software to show data in real time. When I started teaching my only worry was finding the right switch on the sound system to use my iPod instead of the CD.

All this has created a very savvy client and attracted more of the cyclist/triathlete crowd who can see that they can track their training progress indoors with a power meter.

As an instructor, if you don't keep up, you are in trouble as you may get caught out by a rider who knows more about training with power than you do. Do not get complacent as you never know who turns up to your classes.

We often underestimate what our riders can or would be willing to put themselves through in a session, but we can also underestimate their knowledge.

A guy who looked like a rugby player turned up to one of my evening classes on IC7 bikes and sat at the back. I went over and offered my help with the set up, but he said he didn't need it. When he returned a week later, I started chatting with him about his FTP as he was using coach by colour system which was optional in this class.

He said that he had attended a class where in the first two minutes of the warm-up riders were told to do drills that would take them to power Zone 5. They were also told to ride at 130–140RPM which, being quite fond of his knees, he refused to do. He told me: 'That instructor had no concept of technique, energy systems or recovery. I never went back.'

Because of his sports background, this man had a sound knowledge of not only biomechanics but training with power and HR and his knowledge far exceeded the instructor's.

If this guy took another class or two with instructors who do not appreciate the value of education, he may have concluded that we are all just random people who accidentally ended up in a cycling studio with no knowledge to back it up.

I understand that even if you teach indoor cycling, it may not be your main passion or the only class format you teach, but your clients in each of these classes *expect* you to be the *teacher*, the instructor, to know more than they do. If you want to be respected, respect your riders by bringing your best to the table each time.

There are many **CPD courses** that you can attend in person or even take online like ©Stages, ICG® or Spinning®, to name a few. Attending indoor cycling events and Master Instructor rides always boosts my motivation.

Learn to use **online profile building platforms** like Intelligent Cycling®, ©Stages or ICG® Training apps.

When you realise and accept there is so much to learn and improve on in this field, you will keep the excitement going. There is no limit to continuous education.

If you have already followed this advice and need a further challenge, the next chapter should help.

CHAPTER 15
Special Populations

If teaching at regular gyms and studios no longer rocks your boat and you would like to challenge yourself there are options that will push your limits. You can specialise in working with specific populations.

Older riders

I decided to tackle this group first as it is a mostly disputed 'special population' when it comes to indoor cycling.

When you qualify as a group ex instructor, if you want to teach over 50s you should get an 'Older population' qualification. However, when it comes to cycling or indoor cycling this categorisation is pointless. Cycling is a low impact sport so you do not have to worry about modifications, osteoporosis etc., too much. You can make set up adjustments and allow standing breaks whenever necessary but no need to create a special class for a group of 60-year-olds.

Someone asked a question on one of the forums about what ideas others had for an over 50s class and it caused an outrage. Many of us, experienced instructors, are on the other side of 50 or even 60 and there are a few over 70, too. That is the beauty of the stationary bike.

Age in indoor cycling is just a number. As long as you do the health screening as you would do ahead of any class, there is nothing you would teach differently.

Kids

To teach youngsters you may need a special certificate so that you can get insurance. YMCA does a certification to teach kids, but it has nothing to do with a cycling class specifically.

If your gym or studio asks you to teach kids, like 10–14-year-olds, there are a few things to consider:

- Will your insurance cover it?
- What certification will the gym need?
- What bikes does the gym have and do they allow for enough adjustment to accommodate the kids' height?
- Would you know how to teach, get through and motivate a group of 15–20 kids?
- Would you know how to keep an eye on them throughout, so they do not exceed the recommended RPM and risk an injury? (especially when no consoles are present.)

Teaching kids is very challenging so group numbers must be carefully considered. Having an assistant to help would be a good idea.

My friend teaches a group of teenage athletes using Stages bikes and Stages Flight software and that works fantastically. She runs in-class competitions which work like a charm with young boys. Also being able to track their numbers throughout the class helps keeping them focused and disciplined.

It is a great idea if you are up for it and it will mean raising the next generation of indoor and possibly outdoor riders.

Parkinson's Cycling Coach

The path I chose to follow was to obtain a certification to teach indoor cycling to Parkinson's patients. It was a fascinating course and my next mission is to get the project off the ground in London when this type of class is not offered yet. It is not offered anywhere in the UK yet, but this format is very popular and has had a great success in the USA.

Sorting out the insurance cover was a bit tricky as the certification comes from the USA. The only option to get a UK based qualification would require completing a one-year-long university degree which I was not prepared to commit to.

However, there are courses out there that you could check out to see what would keep your fire going. Simply contact the nationally and internationally recognised bodies like REPs (in the UK) and YMCA. They may advise you of university courses they recommend.

The research behind this programme is fascinating as it shows that regular cycling sessions help to improve many of the motor symptoms of PD and motivate the people with PD to leave their houses and form a community. Any physical fitness gains are really a side effect.

Cancer patients

There is no specific course related to this but there are hospitals running or co-running qualification for PTs to become qualified in cancer rehab (at least in London). People recovering from the side effects of chemotherapy and radiotherapy can have balance issues, neuropathy etc., which make walking tricky but once you get them on a stationary bike, they feel secure and can focus on getting some physical activity done which is crucial to their recovery. And just like with Parkinson's patients, this type of class introduces the all-important social factor.

Disabilities: amputees, blind riders, MS, cerebral palsy

You never know who can walk into your next class and even though you cannot be expected to know how to tackle each or any of these scenarios as normal certifications do not delve into them, it is good to give it some thought and pay attention to any discussions between fellow instructors who have this type of riders in their classes.

Amputees

When it comes to amputees, I have had one guy who is an experienced indoor rider but normally doesn't come to my class. His arm is missing from the shoulder socket level. He is incredibly fit and his balance on a bike sitting or standing is great. He rides without any prosthetics.

If I had someone like that coming into a class as a complete beginner, I would spend extra time setting them up and trying to gauge their ability to hold themselves steady on the bike. Ideally, I would like to ask them to come for a 20–30min individual session where we could calmly assess any possible issues and address the weight distribution, balance, and how they would cope with changing resistance. Can they mount and dismount safely on their own?

That would be a perfect scenario, but the truth is that usually a rider like that will come at the last minute to avoid a fuss. They also don't want to be told they cannot attend the class, so they sneak in. I have a girl who is now a regular but initially I had no idea she was missing an arm from the elbow until I was walking around the studio during the class. If they are doing fine and enjoy the class, there is no need to make a big deal out of it.

Blind riders

I taught a fantastic triathlete who is totally blind. He is very attuned to his body since he can only ride to RPE and beat. The classes were led using a coach by colour system but that was of no use to him, so I had to ensure I was totally clear on RPE. In this case however, I knew that the rider was blind as he was brought in by a staff member.

Recently I taught a class on Stages bikes where I refer to the console data quite a lot. There was a lady in the front row who first had a towel over the console. After 15 minutes or so she took it off, but I realised that despite straining she could not read the console. She has never told me about her issue, but I have seen many short-sighted people who don't like riding wearing glasses and then struggle reading the consoles, so I thought this was the case.

After the class I approached her to congratulate her for her hard work and broached the subject of her not being able to see the data and then she told me she was a registered blind. Again, she was a very fit person who was just cross training in preparation for a five-kilometre race with a guide a week later.

Some people may not be very forthcoming with disclosing their issues as they want to be treated the same as everyone else and also worry you may not allow them to take the class if you feel you are not qualified to handle their disability (boy, I hate that word). There is nothing you can do about that. However, once the cat is out of the bag, approach them and explain in a non-condescending way that you can help them make the workout even better or more efficient if you work out a system of cueing that will work for them.

Deaf riders

I have not had a deaf rider in my classes – at least not one I knew of – but I have seen posts on forums from instructors who have. If you ride with a console, the issue is not massive as they can stick to numbers regardless of not being able to hear the music. If your studio has a PIQ system or if you ride with Stages Flight, then there is no issue whatsoever and no extra cues are needed.

Other than that, the rider would mimic your or another rider's leg speed and position in terms of RPM and when it comes to RPE you would need to step up your visual cues. Use your arms when on the bike to cue standing up or sitting down. Use your fingers to count down. Use your facial expression to show the level of exertion. Point to the appropriate body parts to cue form. It would also be a great idea, when you know this rider is coming and when you do not use an overhead display of any kind, to have a class profile printed out for them with sections, RPM, RPE and times highlighted. In the case of deaf riders using apps like ICG Training, Intelligent Cycling or Stages Flight is invaluable.

MS (multiple sclerosis) and CP (cerebral palsy) riders

I have had both in my classes and in both cases had no idea what the issue was and if it wasn't for riding with power meters, I would not have any idea that something was amiss. In both cases the conditions affected one side of the rider's body which meant one side was doing all the work and the other one was there for a ride, pun intended.

The lady with MS struggled a bit on longer intervals and on sprints. Sometimes I felt like she was just holding back. Then after she got to know me a bit more and we built a rapport she explained that some days were better than others but in general as she can only properly push through one side of her body, that side was tiring quite quickly.

In case of the other guy, we were riding Stages bikes which have a power meter on the left pedal crank. Every time I was walking around the studio and his body would be telling me he was high on the RPE scale, like 8–9 out of 10, his console would read 80–90 watts which is very low. He was going guts out and the numbers were pitiful. I have asked him to change the bike a couple of times and tried his bike myself and everything was fine. I was dumbfounded. You see, you need to see him walk a good 20–30 steps to really pick up on one side not performing 100%, but I would only see him do 5–10 steps in the tiny studio.

Finally, after he realised I was hell-bent on working out what the issue was, he told me he had CP that affects his left side and the mystery was solved. As the power is read only from the left crank and his left side does not do much, the readings were super low, so we just worked using the RPE and learnt to not worry about the data much.

As an instructor be prepared that if something does not seem right, even if the riders is not forthcoming with information, do not give up and keep digging. Just let them know that you want to make sure they spend their time safely and efficiently and can improve their fitness and achieve any goals they set themselves.

Diabetes

This condition is more common that we would like to admit. There are different types of it and different ways of managing it that I will not delve into here.

It is crucial that you always ask your pre-screening question: Are you on any medication I should know about? They may not come forward. Their diabetes may be the very reason they came in and now they are worried you may ask them to leave.

I have many diabetics in my classes. One of the fittest riders I have ever had uses the high-tech monitoring system with an implant embedded in his arm that he scans using his mobile phone during the class when he feels things are not going as they should. It's all very bionic.

Some instructors say you should always carry sweets or a sweet drink with you in cases like that. To be honest, if I teach grown-ups I don't necessarily think it is my responsibility to carry these, but it definitely helps to know of the condition so if anything goes wrong and an emergency procedure has to be implemented, you do not waste time trying to work out what the issue might be.

Should you ever refuse a rider taking part in your class?

I think apart from the cases I discussed in Chapter 5 (latecomers or people without any footwear), anyone can take part in an indoor cycling class.

Sports teams – become a coach

If you fancy putting in some serious grafting in terms of education, you have the option to become a British Cycling Coach. There are various levels to the qualification with Level 1 requirement being preparing and teaching a session to grownups outdoors. After Level 3 you can choose if you want to specialise in track, BMX, etc., and then you can start training individuals.

You can try creating a programme yourself (without gaining an official qualification) and delivering it as a private course. I have done it successfully and got a great buzz of it. It was a six week programme in winter, and I will do it again.

You may be approached or you may decide to approach a local sports team that could use indoor cycling as a part of their training. It may be a football or rugby club. They may not require you to be a fully qualified cycling coach as that is only a sideline to their training but they will want you to be able to create a programme, deliver it and show results. Just make sure you can deliver on your promise.

CHAPTER 16
Auditions

Psychology of an Audition. Is it Your Thing?

An audition is a very interesting concept. Even more so an audition for a group ex instructor. I respect gyms and studios who organise auditions and admire those who are not willing to allow you to even cover a class unless they know your credentials, see you teach or have a first-hand recommendation. That being said, I hate attending auditions.

Some people are just not good at auditioning the same way you may really love maths and be good at it but just never do well in exam environment.

I think people who teach more cycling orientated profiles, use periodized programmes and structured rides with one element leading to another, find having to showcase what they can do in three to 10-minutes very challenging.

Some studios have clear requirements: 'Prepare a climb track, include some sprints, in and out of the saddle, show us how you cue and motivate, let your personality shine!' My response to this is: 'in five minutes? How?' One or two track auditions always make me feel like I am underselling myself. Doesn't every instructor know how to ride to the beat and cue people out of the saddle, you ask? If you attended a few auditions, you know that some don't.

The thing that I *know* makes me stand out from the crowd is the attention I give my riders before, during and after the class and the well-thought-out structure of each ride. But I can't show these in two tracks taught in front of a group of other instructors. It's about how I motivate people through a long, 15-minute climb or tempo ride but I can't show it in five minutes.

Another thing when you audition is that you teach a group of fellow instructors. That is why I struggle coming across as my real self and realising my full potential as an instructor in auditions where you sit in front of other instructors who are often just focused on thinking that they are next to take the stage or analysing the performance they had just given. Loads of them just fake the enthusiasm trying to help you. That crowd reacts well to whooping and, 'Are you having fun?!' yells but that's not my style.

I truly believe that auditions should be in front of a real group of riders that could be incentivised by a token of appreciation or a discount from the gym for sitting in. (At least I wouldn't feel bad if I know some riders need their bike set up changed. You don't feel like you can do it to a fellow instructor, right?)

Teaching to 10 other instructors however is still better than teaching to either just a studio coordinator who may just sit on a bike in front of you and not even ride. I have suffered through a few of those. Unless you hold a degree in performing arts, you will struggle. Do I cue imaginary riders' form? Do I look around pretending there are people? Do I ask the imaginary crowd questions? Is that going to bag me a new permanent class or a straightjacket and a place at a secured facility?

These auditions miss the main point: what is the instructor like in interaction with riders? Do they notice someone struggling? Do they keep eye contact? Etc. It would be so much better if the people who want you on board attended one of your normal classes start to finish.

Nevertheless, we must suffer through these whether we like them or not. ICA has a few short articles on auditions but also a more in-depth series that I wrote and parts of which I will use here.

How to Prepare for an Audition

Here is my advice on tackling the dreaded audition. First, it is all about the background checks to decide if you want to audition. Then we will discuss preparing the actual audition. Finally, we will talk about what happens next.

What bikes do they have?

I always start with this one. Not all indoor cycling bikes are created equal. Knowing the brand of the bike will allow you to do some research so you are not thrown off when you walk into the studio. If they have old school bikes with no data and you are used to teaching with metrics, you will need to cue differently. You may also decide NOT to audition at all.

On the other hand, if they have newer bikes with computers or power meters, and you are not familiar with teaching with these tools, you'll have to consider learning how to do so prior to your audition or clarifying if using available data (watts, HR, RPM, calories) is assessed during the audition. Some studios with the newest bikes on the market highlight the fact that new instructors don't need experience on that specific bike as training would be provided. However, this is not a given, so don't assume you will be trained — ask in advance if training is provided.

On bikes with power meters, are you expected to refer to FTP and power zones? Or perhaps you are not supposed to use wattage at all because they haven't been trained on how to use power (or may not care to ever use power)? You don't want to come across as teaching over everyone's head but if this IS your style, will you feel comfortable abandoning it completely?

Learn everything you can about the studio, their culture, and their current team of instructors

Start by checking their website to ensure you agree with their ethos and what they want you to teach. Check their class descriptions and any class videos on their website or on YouTube. You do not want to waste your time if their primary class offerings are not what you are prepared to do or if they go against your certification or standards. At the same time, it will give you an advantage when you show that you have done your research about them.

Check the instructors' bios on their website. Do they list their qualifications? Do they promote the different styles and music tastes of instructors?

Where possible attend a couple of classes with different instructors in different time slots or try to get in touch with someone already teaching there and ask questions. How much focus is placed on proper set-up and technique? Do they value the importance of recovery and variety? How do they express intensity—is it power, heart rate, or perceived exertion? Do instructors tend to teach to the beat? How about variety of music … are all genres welcome or are there restrictions?

In addition to their style and culture, taking classes will give you a chance to see what their demographics are so you can tailor your own audition to suit them. Your approach will differ if you are teaching to mainly millennials or to riders in their 40s or 50s.

Get detailed information about the audition requirements and expectations

Is it just an on-the-bike audition, or will it include an interview?

How long will you have for the audition? Five minutes is much different than 15 or 30.

Do they want you to include a warm-up, cool down, or stretch?

Do they require that you include any specific intensity or terrain, such as intervals, climbing, sprints, etc., or do they just leave it up to you?

Are you allowed to have notes? We discussed how using these may be perceived very differently by different people.

Is it just you auditioning, or will there be many applicants at the same time?

If it's a group audition, will you know the order in advance? You will also know that you cannot do it in your lunchbreak. Also, find out if you are required to stay to the end after your turn. If there are numerous instructors auditioning at the same time, you may be required to stay for up to two hours or more.

The longest one I attended was a full day; unpaid, of course. First, there was a presentation about the studio and its ethics. Next, we had to sit through three tasters of all formats offered by the studio which were delivered by their master instructors. Then after a long lunchbreak during which the studio was used for their regular lunchtime classes, we started the auditions.

Check their address and timetable

Does the schedule suit you? What would the commute be like? If driving, would your desired time slot be subject to rush-hour traffic? If in a big city and you will be using public transportation, are there alternative modes of transport if the trains are cancelled? If this is a lunchtime slot and you still have an office job where you may be held you up extra 10–15 minutes with a last-minute meeting, will you be able to make it to start the class on time?

Find out everything you need to know about the audio and visual systems in the studio

What is the cable connection for music devices? Is the stereo system close to the bike so you will be able to see your device, or is it across the room? Is there a working mic? Will you need your own batteries? If you use Spotify, do they have Wi-Fi, or will you need to download your playlist? Is there a display system (such as Performance IQ) and do they want you to use it? Often studios who have this technology don't want it used during the auditions even if you have the experience. Never underestimate how different it is to teach using bare RPE if you are used to teaching with coach by colour or using PIQ. If suddenly you are expected NOT to refer to power zones or FTP percentage it may really throw you off.

Armed with all your research about your upcoming audition it is time to sit down to prepare your audition. You have been told what they are expecting, both in length and content, so preparing what you will do will be easier.

Putting it all together

Here is where you will use all the intel gathered so far and combine it with your experience plus an added dose of your personality. It is usually best to use an interval profile. Not only is it the most common and popular type of class, but you are also able to put together different combinations of terrain (climbs and flats), cadences (suggestion: limit your cadence to 60 to 100 rpm), and intensities (low, moderate, hard, and very hard). Depending on the length of time you've been given, you can vary your intervals from one to a few minutes (depending on overall audition duration) so you can showcase how you would coach the required intensity differently.

Music choice

With only a few minutes to showcase your skills, it's wise to choose songs that people know. Have you watched *The X Factor*? Sometimes a person in the competition is not the best singer but comes out with a song that everyone knows and can dance to, so it gets the audience going; suddenly a couple of bum notes get overlooked. But if they choose an ambitious Whitney Houston song, the panel is less forgiving. Same with your audition – if you risk a song nobody knows, even if you are excellent at your cueing, the vibe may not be there.

I say this from experience … I once used a song that worked very well in my classes, but taken out of context for a short audition, it failed miserably.

Make sure it's a song that you know extremely well. You need to know where the beat drops so you can use it to build up intensity and time your cueing perfectly. This music cueing skill may give you more points than almost anything else you do in your audition.

As you'll see below, if you are auditioning at a studio or club that leans more toward the 'rhythm' style, choosing popular or new music is more important than it might be if you are showing a more cycling-specific training session.

The elephant in the room …

What if they are more of a 'rhythm ride' type of studio and you are more of a cycling-specific type of instructor? If that is the case and you still decided to audition you can still be successful without compromising your principles.

You must be able to ride to the beat of the music. Select popular songs with differing bpm to show you can match the beat. These classes are usually more varied with more frequent transitions in and out of the saddle (make sure to be on the beat when you move between sitting and standing). On one hand, this kind of presentation is easier to prepare, but your song choice (popular music) will be even more important.

They want to see high energy. That doesn't mean you have to yell, but make sure to engage and make eye contact with everyone in the studio. Even better, try to get everyone to smile and to even yell 'whoop whoop!' as they summit a climb.

In addition to verbal cues, use non-verbal cues to reinforce form and intensity, and use your fingers to count down to the next interval and your hands to indicate in and out of the saddle.

There is still no need to do a single push-up, isolation, or tap-back.

Cycling-specific

If you use a more cycling-specific approach to coaching and you've found a studio that is seeking an instructor like this, congratulations. However, that does not mean you can't borrow the energy from the 'rhythm' world. Remember, we need to combat the myth that this type of class is boring.

First, you can still use the bpm to define cadence – it's not an either/or situation. In fact, it's a wonderful way to give cadence guidelines. However, it will be less likely to be expected, so if that's not your thing and you know it's not theirs, don't worry.

Second, be assertive and powerful. Do not wave the towel over your head if it's not your style but let your personality shine.

For outdoor cycling-oriented auditions, it may get a bit tricky if the audition is really short as it's harder to create a flow to your class with a clear goal. This is where you will need to explain what you would normally do in a full-length class.

However, if you have 15 minutes or more, create a mini profile of a condensed class. Include just enough of a warm-up to explain your objective as if it was a full-length class and leave a short recovery at the end so you can discuss the outcome. A good option is to do a four- to five-minute climb in and out of the saddle with a few accelerations, finishing with a hard push to the summit. Next, add a track of HIIT, making sure you are very clear on intensity by using the metrics available combined with very specific RPE cues. Visualisation cues will be more welcome in this format, as will reminders about good cycling technique.

Be ready for anything

Regardless of the style, be prepared to have your time cut short or to do something on the spot. Again, I'm saying this from experience and from talking to other instructors who have had to pivot at the last minute. They may ask you to cut each song after a couple of minutes or ask you to finish after the second track when you were planning to go out with a big flourish in the last track. It can throw you off, so be ready.

You may hear, 'OK, that's good, just do a hill track now.' For this reason, I suggest you create an audition playlist with a few of your favourite core songs for hills, sprints, short intervals, climbs, or jumps that you can grab at a moment's notice.

Sell yourself from the start

The biggest challenge for any instructor during an audition is to show their unique selling points in a space of only a few minutes. As Jennifer Sage put it in her piece on very short auditions, it is crucial, 'to optimize every second. You need to let them know that you really do know what you are talking about, not just during those three minutes but also during other parts of the class.'

Make sure you are on the ball from the get-go. If there are 10 or more instructors auditioning, I can almost guarantee the time slots will be getting shorter as time progresses. If you waste the first few minutes without showing your teaching skills, you may never get the chance.

Don't forget your setup

As you set up your bike, use this as an opportunity to do a live commentary on the importance of a proper setup. You might be surprised how many instructors do not set their bike up when they get on stage.

Pep talk

As you are on your way to the audition, put yourself in a positive frame of mind. If you were encouraging a fellow instructor, what would you tell them? Now say it to yourself. Go get them!

Then, just before your turn, while the previous instructor is cleaning the bike for you or even as you sit on that bike in front of everyone, close your eyes for a brief moment, take a deep calming breath, and in your head, give yourself some resounding encouragement: *Let's do this! It's showtime!* Then open your eyes, smile, and off you go.

When you get the job! Successful audition – what next?

Congratulations! You got the gig. Now you will need to learn the culture of the club or studio, get to know other staff and the clients you will work with.

There are still a few things you need to ensure happen in a timely manner and a few things you need to be clear about to avoid any possible conflict with management or riders.

Firstly, make sure you get your contract sorted as soon as possible. Make sure you are aware of the notice period (either way). Then get the invoice submission procedures, cut off dates and the payment terms. Make sure you have contact details for anyone to resolve payment queries.

Be clear on how it works with getting a cover for your classes. Is there a pre-approved list you must use, or can you advertise on social media or contact any instructor you know? What about emergency covers?

What is the realm of your responsibility leading to a class and immediately after? Do you need to get an attendance list from reception or collect tokens? What is the policy on late arrivals? What about mobile phone use?

Do you need to ensure the bikes are left in a certain way (handlebars and seats down)? Are you responsible for placing towels and water bottles on bikes before the class starts? There was a boutique studio where I covered a few times, where they expected the instructor to put towels on the bikes before the class, clean all the bikes after the session using spray and cloths provided AND mop the floors?! No extra pay, obviously. They were making savings getting cleaners to come in only at the end of the evening.

Are there any policies on air conditioning or use of fans in the studio and regarding the music volume?

How much time is there between classes? Some places only leave five minutes which is unacceptable and means that everybody runs late which causes unnecessary stress.

Are you expected to provide your own batteries and mic shields or are these in place?

What about promoting your classes on social media? Could you or should you do it? One place I used to teach at made it a requirement to open a twitter account and promote the class heavily there.

You may want to know if there is any regular audit of the classes and whether the clients are encouraged to give regular feedback on the instructors and who gets it. The feedback in a new place will be very important.

Bad case scenario. We are sorry to inform you ... How to deal with rejection

Now onto the other scenario when you do not get the gig. There are times when immediately after the audition you know that this probably is not going to work out. Then if it turns out you were wrong it is a bonus.

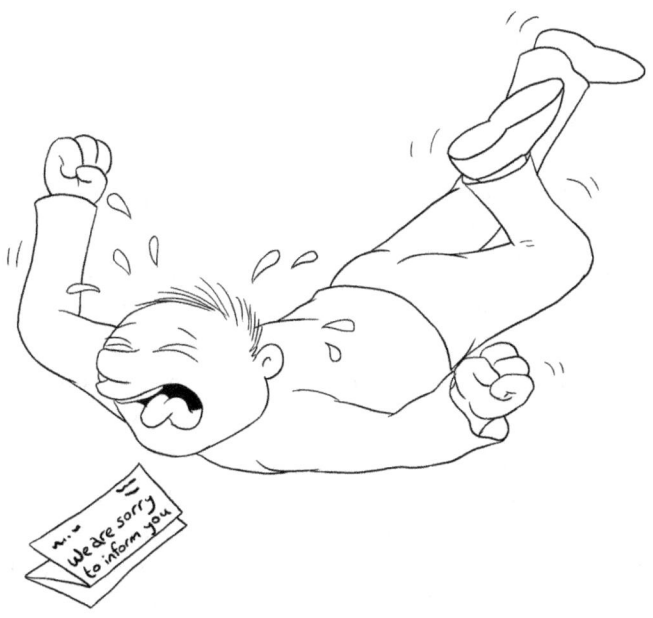

What I hate is when you are convinced you did a good job, you saw other instructors and you know you were right there with the rest of them but it turns out you were not successful.

But let's start from the beginning.

When you attend an audition whether it's an individual one or a group one you will be told that that mysterious 'someone' or 'we' will get back to you. They usually give you the deadline but sometimes they may be a bit vague. If you are told that you will hear back from them, 'in the next few weeks' you need to prepare yourself for not hearing from anyone. Unless you are successful, of course.

I personally hate the lack of respect shown to us as instructors when we gave up a few hours of our day, possibly using a holiday at work, to attend the audition and the studio does not even have the decency to send a generic e-mail saying that it is a no.

My next pet hatred is getting a rejection e-mail without any constructive feedback. If you fail at an audition, or especially at a few, you really want to get to the bottom of it. Is it the cueing, riding technique, music? You want to get better but to do that you need to know where you are going wrong. Therefore, if you only get a one sentence message that you didn't get the job, respond by asking for a more detailed response. However, be prepared for not getting anything for a very long time or ever. That is life.

The truth is sometimes what made them say NO, is not something they are allowed to base their decision on, like your age or looks. Annoying, outrageous but true. Other times the person who gets the gig is the best mate of the studio manager or the person auditioning you. Thankfully I have not witnessed this one often, but I have.

Not getting the job is deflating. Getting a NO a few times is downright depressing, but as I mentioned at the start of this chapter, some people cannot sell themselves in a few minutes even though they are great instructors.

I have been lucky enough that for the first five years I did not attend any auditions. I got all my classes (and I had 14 weekly ones at one point) by word of mouth or through covering a one-off class, then being asked to take on a permanent slot based on clients' feedback.

In the last two years I have attended five or six auditions. I did not get a job from any of them. None. I now react to auditions the same way my body reacts to blood pressure being taken. I know that just sitting in front of that blood pressure monitor is going to make it spike. And it always does. I need to do it three or four times, always getting into a state of meditation first.

You do not get that chance when you audition. Every time I do one, I start doubting my plan, my skills, my choice of music and then it all goes downhill from there. I can teach a class to a group of total strangers, or even ironman competitors, with full confidence yet I have none in the manufactured situation that is a studio audition.

Rejection is not a nice feeling. And if you are passionate about your profession, keep educating yourself and keep filling all your classes yet still cannot be successful in auditions, it is extremely frustrating. I have made a vow not to take part in auditions anymore. It may change in the future. For now, I am done with them. I am in a good position where people (both riders and studio managers around town) know of me and if there is an opportunity to take on a class without the audition process, I can get it.

The main take away is this: if you are not good at auditions that does not mean you are not a good instructor. Just like the fact that you are good at passing exams does not mean you have a thorough understanding of the subject. Find a way to go around it. Make your work ethics and education speak for you.

CHAPTER 17
Studio Logistics

Layout

This may not depend on you at all, but you may be able to give suggestions if you think changing it would benefit the instructor, the riders, or both sides.

Instructor versus riders

It is important that the instructor's bike is visible to as many riders as possible which usually means it is stood on a raised podium. Otherwise I have taught in studios where the riders' bikes are positioned in tiers, like in a theatre so the further the row, the higher it is. This is the best way as everyone can always see the instructor's bike.

It is also best when the instructor is sat in the middle in respect to the group. Some studios position us to the side meaning you keep looking sideways to see everyone which is very uncomfortable.

Instructor vs the sound system and visuals

I am right-handed so when the sound system is to my left, especially if controlled by an iPad, I do struggle a bit, but it is not a major inconvenience. What is much worse is when the controls are behind you or so far that you need to get off the bike every time you want to adjust something.

When teaching with the visuals like Stages Flight, the position of your bike is important to make the full use of all the data on the screen, yet some studios put the instructors with their back to the screen – fair enough, riders are the focus so we need to ensure they can all see it properly and there is always a laptop or an iPad in use with that software showing exactly what the riders can see (and more), yet again in some places it is positioned behind the instructor ... But you must pick your battles.

The point here is, if you think changing the position of any of these would benefit you or the riders, bring it up with the management. It may not be an easy thing to change but it is worth a try.

Temperature in the Indoor Cycling Studio

Oh boy, that is one of those topics that can divide the studios and riders. There are places that keep the indoor cycling studio's temperature quite high on purpose making people believe that this is going to make them sweat more hence make their workout more intense.

Yet if you look at the science of it, and I am talking about doing any kind of intense exercise in a hot and humid environment, it is the exact opposite.

Just to pre-empt here, what follows is not a list of scientific resources and graphs even though you can get into these if you do in-depth research, but as the tone of this book is not scientific, I will present my arguments in layman terms.

There are people who sweat loads and those who don't. Sweating is body's natural cooling system which in some people works more efficiently than in others, therefore when assessing someone's effort level you cannot always rely solely on how much they sweat. The talk test and looking at their form are however invaluable.

Since the studios usually have no windows and with 30 or 40 sweaty riders the air conditioning system is hardly ever coping with maintaining the optimal temperature, the hot air just keeps getting more and more humid as the class progresses and the sweat gets no chance to evaporate. I find it baffling that the studio temperature in all the gyms and studios in London I have ever taught in, is set or limited to 15C which is 59F. If the room is small, maybe 10–15 bikes and empty, this is a nice and cool ambience. Not so much while the people start riding and definitely not if you have 30–40 of them riding for more than 10 minutes.

When the mirrors in the studio steam up less than halfway through the class and I can see riders sitting up for longer periods of time trying to bring their heart rate down, I know it is getting bad.

When you are performing strenuous exercise in a hot and poorly ventilated room, as your core temperature rises, the body needs to protect the internal organs from overheating, so it uses loads of energy on keeping your body's temperature at a safe level. Basically, a lot of energy that could be translated into watts on your bike is instead distributed into that safety mechanism.

Core body temperature has a profound effect on the body's capacity to work. It feels nice to train in warm conditions indoors or outdoors, but there comes a point where the temperature becomes detrimental to your performance.

The optimal body temperature is around 37 degrees Celsius regardless of the ambient temperature or the intensity of your work. To quote Simon Hodder, professor of ergonomics at Loughborough University: 'In the cold you have a strong natural heating mechanism – your exercising metabolism – but it's much harder for your body to cool down than it is to heat up' (www.cyclist.co.uk/in-depth/905/how-does-hot-weather-affect-your-cycling-performance).

Research also shown that if you are used to doing an FTP test outdoors and then ride one in a closed room with just air conditioning and a fan, your results may differ by a significant margin as so much energy is diverted into keeping the body temperature constant.

How hot is too hot?

I am not able to see what the actual temperature of the room is, but a tell-tale sign is when the floor is so sleek with humidity that it resembles a shiny ice-rink. When that happens, I always report it to the management as it is a serious health and safety issue.

This becomes a very serious issue if you have pregnant riders, as overheating is the only serious risk factor when they take an indoor cycling class.

One place where I teach a few classes a week (at the time of writing) we have an industrial fan in the front, and I spend quite some time moving it (it does not turn to change directions) so everyone gets some benefit.

Fans as a Solution

Unfortunately, the guidelines on the preset air conditioning are unlikely to change, even though I would love to learn how they were set. If the air conditioning is in place, working, but just not coping, it is important to reiterate the importance of hydration. Adding some fans in strategic places may be a game changer, as well.

If the air conditioning is broken more radical solutions may be needed like opening any existing windows and keeping the studio door open. These may not always be possible as the loud music may be disturbing people on the gym floor or outside on the street. However, I value the safety of my riders more than an upset receptionist or a PT so I will make a point of bringing it to management's attention that the sooner they fix the fault, the sooner the door will remain closed.

I also tend to tailor the choice of my profiles to accommodate the faulty air conditioning. I favour steady state efforts, with most of the class in the saddle to avoid spikes in heart rate. I also choose long tracks so I can let my riders get on with it and then I ask people who are running out of water to wave their bottle in the air so I can collect it and refill it for them.

Battle of the fan

We have all been through this as instructors: 'Please turn the fan on!', 'Why is the fan not on? 'Why is the fan on?! It's cold!!!' 'OMG it's freezing, please turn it off!' (eye roll.)

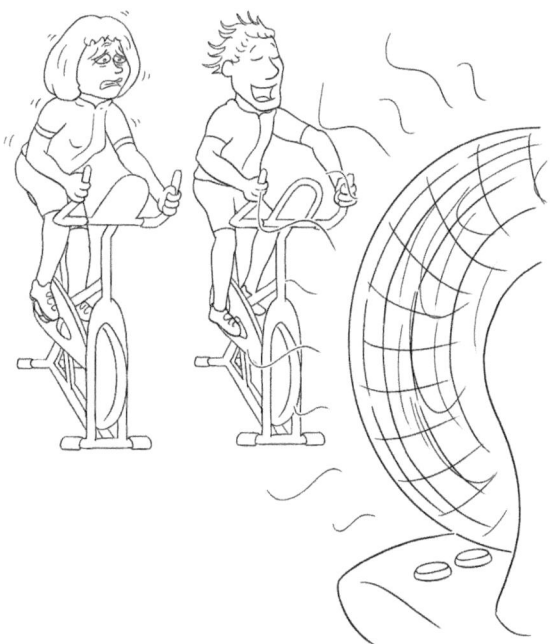

If I can, I do not switch the fans on until the warm-up is over as some of them are indeed powerful and can be very loud. Unfortunately, some are positioned in a way that once the class starts, you cannot get into them without disturbing some riders.

Important thing to say if you use fans is to make it clear to people as they choose their bikes: 'Please note that if you sit close to a fan, it will be turned on once we start'.

Working with power data helped the penny drop for many in terms of understanding the detrimental effect of high temperature in the studio on the results. People can now see that the hotter the studio the harder the workout is a lie. While the RPE goes up, the power drops.

To sum up – when it comes to indoor cycling, keep it cool.

CHAPTER 18

Gym Wear

What to wear? Advice for New Riders

I bet some of you have just thought: 'Is she serious?! But that's obvious!' I am also inclined to think that those who thought that have not been teaching for long. What have I seen over the years to prompt me to devote a separate chapter to this subject?

Footwear

I have already talked about it in Chapter 5. I have seen flip flops, barefoot running things and just plain socks. Always advise the riders to wear comfortable trainers ideally with a sturdy sole that won't bend too much. Keep the shoelaces short or tucked in.

Tops

Indoors I would advise against cotton T-shirts but if they are just starting, it is not a big problem. The issue with cotton clothes is that they get soaked with sweat that doesn't evaporate. The top then just sits heavy on the skin and when they cool down, it makes you feel freezing cold and unpleasant. Wicking fabrics are the best.

I suggest wearing a couple of layers so the long sleeve top can be taken off after the warm-up.

Bottoms

Some people who have not done much cycling in their life come wearing tiny shorts. This is *never* comfortable, regardless of your size, if the shorts are skimpy your bare skin will rub against the saddle and it is a big no-no. If a beginner turns up sporting these, I do mention it to them and give them permission to leave early if it gets uncomfortable and advise them to wear longer shorts or leggings next time.

The other extreme are full length sports bottoms with flares. Thankfully, there is no danger of the trousers getting caught up in the chain as they would on an outdoor bike, but I still advise to wear shorter variety or leggings.

Headwear and other religious garments

I tend to worry a bit about women who come to classes with headscarves, long sleeves and long bottom outfits but only if the air conditioning is not sufficient. Just advise them to drink plenty.

I once had to set up a lady wearing a full burka on a Stages bike. It was almost impossible as there was fabric everywhere. I did my best, but I did tell her that she should not take a class wearing it. This was at a studio launch so it was not followed by a class and thankfully they do offer women only classes where they can take these garments off.

How to Deal With Wet Cycling Shoes?

Cycling shoes are a real game changer in terms of quality of your workout. They make all the difference when you increase resistance and work out of the saddle. You don't have to worry about loose shoelaces or your foot moving in the pedal cage. They are essential if you have big feet.

Just like with trainers, there is a wide variety of cycling shoes, some more breathable than others. People who ride outdoors may prefer their shoes to be as waterproof as possible but when buying a pair for indoor cycling only, think about having as much ventilation as you can.

Take care of your shoes by airing them to allow them to dry after each workout as soon as you get home from the gym, take the shoes out of your bag. You can leave them somewhere warm and dry indoors or if you can, take them outside and leave them in a warm and sunny spot.

If they start smelling nevertheless, use an anti-odour spray that you can get in pharmacies or even shoe shops. Some boutique studios where you can rent cycling shoes use very effective sprays after each use.

Running and cycling shops also sell plastic balls that are odour eaters. You just pop them into the shoes when you get home, or use an old school method like baking soda or dryer sheets.

If you had a particularly long session in a hot studio, your shoes may feel soaked inside. Use an old newspaper tightly balled inside overnight to soak up the moisture.

How to Ensure Your Kit Does Not Smell?

Wash it. Simple as that. Wash it. Every use. No, taking your top off to let it dry is not enough. The fact that you walked home from the gym and your top and leggings dried off doesn't change the fact that it got sweaty and the bacteria is there just waiting to be soaked up again to strike with the deadly stink. Reheated sweaty kit gives off a punchy odour that can only be rivalled by the one of a kit washed but not fully dried, or not washed at a high enough temperature. It is simply vile.

You must wash your gym clothes as soon as you can but if you don't have enough to do a wash that often, then try to get your used kit to dry as much as you can before putting it in a washing basket for a couple of days until you have a full load. If you leave your wet clothes in the basket, they become chemical waste.

Another tip, if you bring your gym clothes back home in those single use plastic bags that are available in the changing rooms, make sure you take them out of those before you put them in the washing basket. Otherwise wet and hot clothes in a tied-up bag festering for a couple of days will develop their own ecosystem that will require a double wash.

Almost a year ago I bought a gym bag that has a separate pocket for shoes and a built-in bag for wet clothes. It has been a game changer and it has reduced my use of single use plastic bags by 100%. It is big enough for two full sets and then some. And I never forget to take it with me as it is permanently attached to the bag.

When it comes to washing your gym clothes, there is a school of thought that says you should not use fabric softener on wicking materials as it stops them from performing their function. I still use it. I do not use high temperatures.

Take the washing out as soon as you can and let it dry fully. If you have an outside space, use it.

I live in London in a flat with no outside space or balcony and we have electric heaters which you cannot use for drying clothes on so I opted for a heated dryer that fits a full load of washing, uses very little electricity and folds back to sit behind the living room door when not in use. When you cover it with a bed sheet, duvet cover or a special cover that you can buy with it, it will dry everything overnight. I could not recommend it enough.

CHAPTER 19

Hygiene in the Studio

I have consciously separated this issue from the previous chapter when we talked about what to do to keep your clothes smelling fresh. Here I will raise the issue of personal hygiene and the smell people's bodies can give off, making everyone around them question their will to live. I am talking about that kind of BO that makes people around gag and unfortunately it happens more often that we would like.

What To Do With a Stinky Rider?

This is quite a big problem if you find yourself riding next to someone like that in a stuffy, hot and humid studio with possibly a fan blowing that fragrant combo right in your face. It can put you off the whole workout and I have people in my classes leave, only to tell me later that this was the reason for their abandoning the class.

This is a very awkward issue to raise and you may not feel that you know how to approach it at all, let alone without singling anyone out. As an instructor I have smelled bad BO when walking around during the class but also right at the point of helping people set up, which does not bide well for when their body temperature rises and sweat comes out.

In my experience, the culprits often wear the wrong clothing, old and worn out shoes or baggy jogging bottoms. The issue is sensitive as these riders may not be able to afford new shoes and face the choice of either wearing the old smelly things or not coming to the gym. These riders often seem unaware of the problem.

Another thing you may want to consider is that some people have an issue with a bad BO despite trying to remedy it, but I strongly believe they make up a tiny fraction of the worst offenders.

How to tackle the issue then?

If you don't know where to start, talk to the management and bring to their attention the fact that other riders are complaining and that it affects the overall attendance. If they are not prepared to help, you may have to take the bull by the horns and kick up a stink, pun intended, about the importance of personal hygiene in a spin studio environment at the start and at the end of each class.

If the message is not getting through you may want to say that the problem is getting serious and you can smell it when you walk around the studio. Ultimately though, if that person does not get the drift or refuses to acknowledge the problem, you have only two choices: confront them directly or you may have to let it go and have the attendance drop, as you can't stop someone's gym membership based on their BO. At least as far as I know.

Cleaning the bikes

This topic makes me really agitated as there are so many gyms and studio managers that still do not understand the importance of keeping the bikes clean and maintaining them on a regular basis. They spend hundreds of thousands of pounds on state-of-the-art bikes and … that's it. Job done.

Every bike type comes with a manual that includes the description of a cleaning routine and maintenance log that should be printed out and followed. I have yet to see a place that does that.

Some gyms are fantastic and have a team of cleaners walking in as soon as the class ends to wipe the bikes and mop the floors. Others expect the riders to clean up the bikes after they use them. That is fair enough provided they are equipped with either cleaning sprays and paper towels or wet wipes. Unfortunately, it is a common occurrence that none of these are available.

You can buy a Ferrari but if you don't do the MOT on it or keep changing the oil etc., it will break. On average, a spin bike in a busy studio gets used about 20 hours a week. That equals buckets of salty sweat falling all over the exposed bike parts and inside the handle bars stems. If they get no proper chance to dry off and never see a drop of lubricant the crust of sweat and snot just builds up until the bike is rendered useless. It beggars belief how gym and studio managers fail to see this.

As a rider, it is only polite to wipe any bodily fluids from your bike as much as you can, unless the studio makes it obvious that it does it for you. However, if you see that the gym floor does not get washed or the bike stands just grow moss or other fungi, make sure you, as a paying client, complain to the management using proper channels.

CHAPTER 20
Say WHAT?!

If you have read this book from the beginning, you know it is not a scientific publication but more of a chronicle of life experiences. If you are starting from this chapter then you will get a general gist of the tone of the whole book.

I decided to finish with a few topics and real-life scenarios that you as an instructor will encounter sooner or later. These are the kind of questions or statements that will stop you in your tracks unless you thought about them beforehand. Being ready to deal with these gems of scenarios will earn you a Bad Ass Instructor badge.

Please note the topics below are in no specific order as some of them are so random they do not fit in any box.

Farting

This is a very touchy subject. Farting is a bodily function that does happen to all of us. If we are lucky there is no smell to go with it. In a closed studio filled with hot bodies and humid air a person may let off one. It happens, but that is not what I am talking about here. I am talking about having a serious offender who annihilates anyone within a five-metre radius.

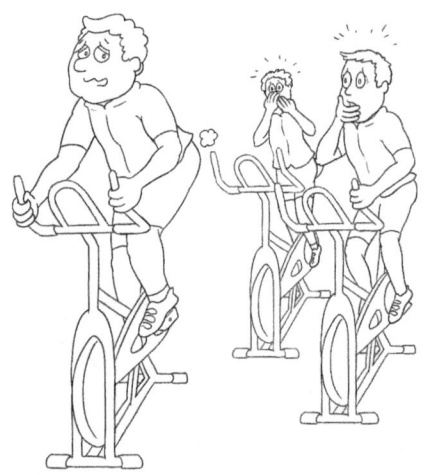

We had this issue in one of my gyms. At the beginning I thought I was the only one who noticed. I would smell it when I was walking around the studio teaching off the bike. But then people started talking about it after classes and so did other instructors. 'Who does it?!' was on everyone's lips. Finally, as it was happening in almost every class and it was bad enough to make us gag and our eyes water, we as instructors had to address it. One of the members even brought in an air freshener and put it right in the front of the studio and said he was not afraid to use it next time the smell wafted towards him.

When it happened again, I turned down the music and said: 'Whoever is doing the farting and thinks they are getting away with it – you are NOT. We can all smell it and it is vile. You have got to stop!'

It was harsh, but necessary. Funnily enough, it stopped after this intervention so clearly the person was in fact able to hold it in, just thought nobody else could smell it as nobody's was saying anything.

Smoking Right Before the Class

A few years ago, a rider came up to ask me: 'What is the latest I should have a cigarette before the spin class?' I am not kidding.

I also had a new rider who came up asking me to help her set up her bike. I followed her and then it hit me – the stench of cigarettes on her clothing and on her breath. She clearly just had a cigarette before coming into the studio. It was an awful experience for me and the riders sitting right next to her.

When the following week I saw her smoking outside the gym I said: 'This is not going to help your performance, is it?' I know it's not my job to make people stop smoking but just like with farting, if it affects people sitting around the offender, you need to raise it.

You can do it by addressing the whole group before the class saying that it just spoils the experience for everyone in the vicinity so all you ask is that the riders do not smoke for at least 20 minutes before they enter the studio and use a chewing gum to freshen their breath.

Lady Bits Issues

It is no secret that indoor (or outdoor) bike saddles are *not* comfortable. There are various types of saddles and when it's your outdoor bike, you can shop around and find the most comfortable one. When you attend cycling classes, you must live with whatever saddle the bike has.

The topic I will raise is the effect saddles can have on women, mainly because I am a woman and other women have come up to me asking for advice. Guys have not. I assume it's because the topic is sensitive rather than they find the saddles soft and comfy.

Firstly, it's about the newbies. I do make a point of saying that when you start taking cycling classes, your bum will hurt, after each one, for a couple of days. I remember that when I started, I wanted to take more classes but after a Monday class I could not sit on a bike on Wednesday. It was so painful that even if I did turn up, I had to leave after 10–15 minutes.

I tell new riders that beginnings are tough but once you get into the rhythm of taking two or three classes a week regularly, your bum gets immune to it (more or less).

To maximise the comfort (or minimise the discomfort) it is important to set the rider up properly paying attention to the saddle fore and aft.

Explain that riding too fast with little resistance will make them bounce which, in turn, will make the bum hurt even more.

Suggest that they buy a gel saddle cover or even padded shorts if the discomfort means that they are put off taking classes altogether.

Whether they wear padded shorts or normal ones, women often get bad problems with their front bits, for lack of better wording. Extreme chaffing can even cause tears in the skin. The general advice on padded shorts is **not** to wear underwear with them but I spoke to a women's health specialist who said even with normal leggings or shorts when cycling, women should not wear knickers. I tend to disagree. But if you are having issues you should try both ways and see what makes it better. Just like with outdoor riders, a chamois cream may be a good solution.

If it gets very painful you may need to take a break and see your GP who can prescribe medication. You then let things settle and heal before you come back.

You will notice that beginner women riders tend to sit up or stand up more than men, simply to relive the pressure so be understanding.

Social Butterfly (Using Phone In Class)

Technology – can't live without it but it's also a curse of our times. The use of mobile phones in spin classes seems to be causing a lot of discussion when in my opinion it should not. Would you use it in a swimming class? What about a boxing class? Body pump? No? Then I guarantee you will survive 45 minutes on a bike. The fact there is a space on a stationary bike you *can* put your phone on, does not make it *necessary* to use it.

Just to clarify, I am not a mobile Nazi – if you are using an app to track your power or your HR, I do not mind when it is in your field of vision. If, however you plan to check your e-mails, news or update Instagram, you need to do it before we start the class or after it's finished.

'But you cannot make people give up their phones! What if something important happens and someone needs to contact them?'

And how did we all cope before 2005? There were people taking gym classes and mobile phones were not omni present. Seeing the screen light up with every new alert will distract you and those around you. Make these 45 or 60 minutes all about you and your workout. If there is an emergency, people can contact the gym.

How do you make people give up their phones?

I announce it clearly before the class starts: 'Take the last photo for your Insta while you still look good and then put the phones on the floor or face down on the bars. You cannot get a workout and check the social media at the same time.' If despite that I catch someone using the phone I turn the music down and ask them to stop.

When I hear instructors' arguments that, 'we don't know what is happening in people's lives,' and therefore we should allow them to do what they like, my blood boils. We don't know what is happening in the lives of the other 30 people in the same studio who came to get a workout and not to get distracted by a glowing screen and someone next to them sitting up typing a message or even worse, talking on their phone during the class. Do you have the same thoughts when someone on a bus or a train plays loud music through their phone or has a very loud conversation for 20 minutes? It's a group exercise environment and selfish rules do not apply. Respect the people around you.

Caveat: I always allow people who may be on call, like doctors or duty solicitors, to have their phone where they can see it but in my experience people who legitimately need them, rarely use them in class. They just get off and leave the studio to answer that important call.

When you use an app tracking your workout etc put your phone in airplane mode and the problem is sorted.

Will The Real Slim Shady, Please Stand Up?

Once I was teaching at a place for a few weeks. A gentleman in his late 50s walked in and proceeded to set up his bike with his saddle at the lowest setting. He must have been around 5–6". I went up to help him and point out the set-up issue to which he said: 'Oh, it's because I don't use the saddle. I do the whole class standing'.

You should have seen my face. I turned around to pick up my jaw off the floor and then I went back to him and said: 'Sorry, did you say you want to ride a 45-minute class out of the saddle?' He said that was indeed his intention as he found sitting extremely uncomfortable and all other instructors allow him to do it his way. He would only get off once or twice to top up his water bottle. He explained that cycling classes were his way of tackling blood pressure and weight issues. He did not like any other exercise classes.

Since I was a new instructor at this place, I decided to give it a go and see him ride. You see I thought maybe he was an amazing rider who could ride with proper technique for that long standing. Suffice to say, once we started it was a car crash: no resistance, locked out elbows, locked knees, mashing the pedals etc and as a result there was no cardiovascular benefit. There was not a bead of sweat in sight, no heart rate elevation.

I walked up to him a few times, but he would not accept my advice so against my professional instincts I decided to stop correcting him and ignore him completely, focusing my attention on the rest of the group instead.

When my final class at that gym came, he was the only person who turned up. I had to think on my feet – doing speed work or intervals was pointless as he was only going around 45–50RPM for the duration of any class, so I went with hills. I also moved my bike next to his, so he had a mirror on the left and me on the right. I turned the music down a bit and took off the microphone.

Usually 1:1 classes are a great opportunity to put somebody through their paces but that would not work here so I suggested something else: 'How would you feel if we did two songs on the bike and then to give your legs a break, we would do some core work on the floor?' Thankfully he agreed.

I wish I could tell you that he got it and climbed to the beat, but I can't. After months of switching off during classes he just could not or would not ride to the beat and continued with is 45–50RPM on low resistance despite me huffing and puffing next to him, albeit a bit over the top to get the point across.

But when I got him to do some planks, Russian twists, screen wipers etc on the floor, boy did his HR go up! He was getting on that bike to get some rest … 45-minutes flew by and he worked up some serious sweat. A combo class like that would be a game changer for him. He was a classic example of a person thinking that getting on a bike is a cardio workout regardless of what they do when they are on it.

I did not want to put it too bluntly that he was getting absolutely nothing from the classes the way he was riding them, since this was the only thing getting him out of the house and into the gym so at least he got extra steps in – hopefully he didn't drive there.

To sum up, riding out of the saddle for more than a minute at a time is to the detriment of riders' technique, whether they acknowledge it or not. The truth is riders like standing up as (apart from bum break) it makes them feel they are working harder due to heart rate elevation – provided they are riding at a sufficient RPM. The RPE is high but the actual power output and, as a result, calories burnt are low.

I used to teach a six-minute climb suggesting the riders should try and stay out of the saddle as much as possible. Until I saw a class taught that way from a perspective of an observer and saw the effect on riding technique of 90% of the group after the first two minutes. I don't do that anymore.

Spinning Won't Make You Fit

This is in a way connected to the previous point. Many PTs claim just that and try to discourage their clients from attending cycling classes. This statement gets me really fired up so I will devote quite a bit of attention to it since it throws up a few statements you are likely to hear from people who argue that indoor cycling is not a useful type of exercise.

Back in 2015 I came across an article that was linked to one of the indoor cycling instructor forums. The title was *'Spinning Probably Won't Make You Fit and Here Is Why'*. Understandably it caused quite a stir amongst all the instructors.

I have come across this statement a few more times since then and it's is something you hear quite often from personal trainers.

The article made a few points to allegedly prove why indoor cycling would not give you fitness gains like getting a PT or lifting weights would. It was based on an interview with a PT Brian Nguyen who as a 'trainer to Mark Wahlberg' should (according to the publication) be treated as an authority in fitness. I will deal with the main points in the next few paragraphs as you will hear these statements repeated by other PTs or even new clients.

> *'Spinning is tough. After an hour of pedalling at high speed, you've probably left a puddle of sweat on the floor under your bike. (...) The classes are fun, and the routines can easily lead to the assumption that participants get a great workout.'*

Anyone who has taken a properly structured indoor cycling class with a qualified and educated instructor, particularly a class based on power zones and using bikes with power meters, will ask: are we talking about the 'dance-on-the-bike-out-of-the-saddle-with-half pound weights' type of class or are we talking about a class based on power? Because the latter involves much more than 'pedalling at high speed/. In fact, the 'speed' or RPM may not be that high at all.

If, however, you refer to classes advertised as a full body workout using weights, resistance bands or other modifications not based on science, then I wholeheartedly agree. But please, Mr PT, do not put us all in the same bag. I have seen plenty of rubbish PTs in action, yet I will not generalise that having a PT is pointless.

> *'Spinning produces similar effects in the body as jogging. (…) Once you finish a spin class, your body no longer burns calories.'*

This part got me really peeved. Jogging? I used to jog. I lost a bit of weight, gained some muscle but the results were not mind blowing. I also never got out of breath, my legs never turned to jelly, nor have I had issues walking up or down the stairs after a jog, however long. (Apart from the six and a half hour Edinburgh marathon which as you can gather from the time it took me to complete it, I did jogging).

What classes has this dude taken, if at all, to make such a statement?!

If I were to give an 'expert opinion' the way this guy did, I would say that even a session with a PT using weights etc has the same effect as the spin class he refers to. How? If you have a bad trainer who gives you weights inadequate to cause muscle overload. What kind of PT would do that? A bad one. And I have seen a few of those. Would I say in an interview with a paper that PT sessions won't make you fit? No, I would however advise you to choose your PT carefully. Same goes about your indoor cycling class. It may take you a while before you find a class that suits your needs. Ask about the instructor's qualification. Question the techniques they ask you to use or not use and listen what they base their answers on.

And what about the part about the effects of a spin session lasting only until you get off the bike? I really question the fitness qualifications of this guy. Whatever exercise you choose cycling, running, swimming, etc you can do them at different intensities depending on your goals: just getting off the sofa, endurance, strength, HIIT etc. Based on the intensity you would expect different outcomes. Would you tell a track runner that since 'jogging' has no fitness benefits their sprint track sessions are useless? Apples and oranges … If every indoor cycling class involved pedalling at the same tempo for 45-minutes who on earth would keep doing them?

I am about to say something here to Brian that may require him to sit down first: you can even do a TABATA session on a bike! I am serious! Not that I would recommend this type of workout to a general population group, but I hope you get my point.

How long your metabolism remains elevated for following an indoor cycling class will depend on the duration, intensity and (as explained in the book *'Roar'* by Dr. Stacy Sims) whether you are a man or a woman.

I am convinced that this guy either took one class in his life, and it wasn't a good one, or he is basing his 'expert' opinion on hearsay.

Now onto the big guns. Brace yourselves:

> 'Spinning doesn't build muscle. (…) Cycling never makes your body gain lean body mass, and that's the thing that burns fat. At the end of the day, metabolism isn't improved on a bike.'

First, the **reference** to spinning isn't exactly true but Mr Nguyen goes beyond that and refers to cycling in general. Let me make something clear at this point: if you only do cycling classes a couple of times a week and no work off the bike, no, you will not build muscly legs and definitely not the upper body. However, if your classes are challenging various skills including muscular strength then you will see a difference. Maybe not as fast or dramatic as training with weights and doing loads of squats and lunges but you will.

If you check out pictures of Marcel Kittel, Chris Hoy (when he was still racing) or Jason or Laura Kenny you will see what I am talking about. Yes, these are extreme examples of professional track cyclists, but Mr Nguyen referred to 'cycling' in general. These guys spend hours building their strength off the bikes but to say that working on the bikes gives them no benefit is a bit much.

'Spinning doesn't give you individual progression.'

It used to be true, but the technology has moved in leaps and bounds, and more and more studios have bikes with power meters, so riders are able to test their fitness using a whole array of tests and then retest periodically to measure the progression. There are many software packages that analyse your training sessions outdoors and indoors like Training Peaks, for example. I will give the guy the benefit of the doubt though as the interview was done in 2015 and indoor cycling has become a different animal since then.

If he is happy to tar everyone with the same brush, I had a PT once (and have seen others) who did not do any measurements before we started working together so no fitness test, flexibility, body fat or others. Nothing whatsoever. Every session we would go on a piece of machinery and he would make no notes of my load so from week to week he had no idea if I was progressing at all. I cannot go on record saying that all PTs are like that.

'Spinning reinforces common injuries.'

Cycling indoors or outdoors involves sitting and we as modern humans do enough of that already, but it is also the best low impact activity, next to swimming, that can help with many health problems and is often used in physiotherapy.

I would like to educate Brian about bike fit. I have witnessed many times a PT bringing their client into the studio to do a warm-up or an interval session and not paying any attention to the bike set up. By doing that they were not only reducing the potential benefit of the session, the client's power output as well as putting their client at the risk of injury because of incorrect bike set up.

Any good indoor cycling instructor will ensure the rider's set up will minimise discomfort and prevent pain. However, the bike set up on its own will not prevent a possibility of an injury if excessive RPM is used, meaning the rider pedals too fast to control the speed of his legs or excessive resistance is used putting unnecessary stress on joints and lower back. Same goes for very low cadences with heavy resistance. For those reasons, guidance needs to be followed and all recognised certifications state these clearly.

To sum up Brian doesn't know much about indoor cycling when he says:

> *'When done on its own, your results from spinning will likely fall short of your expectations.'*

It all comes down to the same principles in all kinds of workouts, PT sessions and indoor cycling included: setting a SMART goal, commitment in achieving it, measurement of progression and testing, paired with the appropriate nutrition.

I Don't Want To Use Much Resistance, So I Don't Get Bulky

If I could get one pound each time I hear a woman tell me that in a class, I would be able to go on a holiday to Australia. It is not that easy, ladies! This is usually the answer I get to my suggestion the woman in question should indeed increase resistance to avoid a concussion due to excessive bouncing in the saddle.

I follow up with a question: 'How many classes do you do a week?' and the answer is always one or two. I wonder where the notion that a random indoor cycling class will result in building strong and muscular legs comes from. I suspect some of the self-made so called Insta-Fitness-Gurus are partly to blame when they spread their unfounded pearls of wisdom ranging from, 'indoor cycling will make you bulky,' to 'spin will make you lose muscle – don't do it!'

I always send these people to look at photos of competitive road cyclists, like Chris Froome and track cyclists like Chris Hoy in his heyday. I point out that cycling as a sport does not have the same outcome for everyone. I also ask if they really think that Sir Chris Hoy got his powerful legs from riding his bike or would the hard-core resistance training have anything to do with his physique.

In all my years of teaching I have never seen anyone bulk up from indoor cycling alone. That remains wishful thinking for many who prefer cycling to weight training.

I had a girl once tell me that she has put on weight since she had started *one* spin class a week about two months earlier. I could not argue that as I did not see her stats before and after. One thing I pointed out to her was being mindful of what and how much she was eating post-class. A hard-core spin class makes you hungry, so you fuel up afterwards often with the attitude of, 'I worked my ass off I now deserve a pizza!' Yet the calorie number you burn on that bike may not be as high as you would hope, especially if you rely on technology basing the numbers purely on your HR or believe in fairy tales, some places try to sell you in saying that you can burn 1,000 in 45 minutes (while using 0.5 kg hand weights for a part of that).

Be careful of what, how much and when you eat. Simple as that. You cannot outride a bad diet.

When you agree to cover a class and the regular instructor sabotages it

What do you do when your holiday is coming up and you know you need to get someone else to teach your classes? What is your or your studio's etiquette? Do you tell you riders or keep them in the dark until they turn up to find someone else in front of them?

There is one gym where we have been instructed not to let riders know when we would be away. I assume it stems from the fact that quite a few people may choose not to turn up if their regular instructor is away. This means less income for the studio and it's not that nice for the cover instructor who was told this was a busy class and then only has a handful of riders turn up.

I think letting people know you will be away – especially if it is for more than an isolated class – is better. Whenever I can I ask the instructors my riders gave me good feedback on previously, to cover my classes. I look for instructors who have similar style to mine. However, this may not always be possible.

When I have no other choice but to accept an offer from an instructor I do not know, I always give them a lowdown of what my style is about and what the people are used to, making the fact that I do not include upper body moves a priority. I do not expect anyone to change their style to cover two or three of my classes but I think it is only fair to both the instructor and the riders to make the expectations clear.

If I don't know much about the person who agreed to cover or I know their style is very different from mine, I address my regulars during the last class before my leave asking them to not skip the class and still work as hard as they normally do. I also say that if they are asked to perform a move that they feel is not effective or 100 percent safe, to just stay in the saddle and stick to the basics.

I then ask for the feedback when I get back so I know if they are happy for me to use that instructor again or would they rather I didn't. Some gyms arrange covers for their instructors so I have no decision or knowledge of who will be coming in to teach my groups.

I would never refer disrespectfully to another instructor or use the opportunity to tell my riders not to come in when I am away. Unbelievably, I have heard of instructors who do just that. I think this may stem from their own insecurities. But remember about Karma.

The Turf Wars – This Is My Bike!

Humans are territorial, and at the risk of sounding ageist, the older they are the more territorial they get. I have a regular rider who will simply not take a class if 'her' bike is taken. I may roll my eyes at that until I remember that I used to do the same as a rider … I had two bikes that were positioned just right to alleviate my anxiety: you could see the clock if you wanted to, but it was not in your face. You could see yourself in the mirror if you looked sideways, but it wasn't in front of you and they were in the last row, so nobody was behind me. I had been known to leave the room if they were taken. Please do not judge me as I tried other bikes, but they didn't feel right. I called it force of habit, but my sister blamed my old age (I was 30 at the time).

As an instructor you are not obliged to get involved in the turf wars unless someone came in first, put their stuff on the bike and maybe left to get water only to find someone else sitting on that bike on their return. This behaviour is unacceptable, and you should get involved if asked for intervention.

I have a great bond with my regulars and they follow me on social media so sometimes they send me a message before the class that they may be coming at the last minute and would I please save their regular bike for them, which I do not mind at all. And my most particular rider? Even if she doesn't ask, if I see her name on the list, I do save her the bike. And if someone else had already sat on it, I have been known to politely ask if they wouldn't mind getting a different one – only if they want to, there is no obligation. I am nice like that.

Panic At The Studio – When Fitness Gets Scary

Fitness means different things to different people and getting fit can be a daunting prospect. Whether people turn to fitness due to media pressure or following a warning from their GP telling them their blood pressure and cholesterol are through the roof or that their BMI number means they are now categorised as obese, the main thing is that they take their first step by signing up with a gym or decide to try out a class.

If they feel particularly brave or highly motivated, they may sign up for a cycle class even though the flashing lights, loud music and the amount of Lycra on display can raise their heart rate before they even touch a bike.

I want to make you, instructors, aware of how scary working at high intensity can be, particularly in an indoor cycling studio. If you take a general HIIT class, you may simply walk out if it gets too much. No big deal. But in your first class on an indoor bike where you are not sure how to release your feet safely, it is dark, the bikes are closely packed, the music is pumping, it is easier said than done.

These people have found enough courage to make their way into the studio, but they may have never done intensive cardio work. They may know what to expect in terms of moving their legs fast, they know they may be expected to stand up and sit down throughout but what about in physiological sense?

I have had a few riders that were truly petrified of going anaerobic or at VO2 max intensity, of working hard enough for the legs and lungs to burn, for the HR to soar, to experience the level of exertion when you don't have much more left to give. Scrap that, they were scared as soon as their breathing would start to change, and they could feel their HR increase slightly.

Make no mistake, we are not confusing a lack of commitment or laziness with an actual fear of never having been in a self-induced state of this level of exertion.

As instructors, we don't know what brought them to this point – prior experience or lack thereof. The question is, are we willing to take them on this journey? If we are then there is some serious 1:1 work needed, which means us getting off the bike for certain parts of the workout when that personal attention is needed.

How do you recognise that this is what the rider is experiencing? It is not easy to spot as these riders look just like you and me. They do not have to be obese, of certain age or sex.

The eyes and the face will be the give-away showing they are scared but some of them may verbalise their fear when given a chance – if you ask them how they feel. For some people just getting a bit breathless brings on a level of fear comparable to facing a bungee jump. I have seen riders practically hyperventilating, tearing up and having a mild panic attack.

How do you handle such situations? First, it is about recognising the issue and then being tactile in letting the person know that you know, understand and can help them.

Giving the rider control is of utmost importance. You need to make them aware that whatever you ask the group to do, they can take it at their own pace whether it is adjusting the intensity or the length of the interval. If the plan is to do a series of, let's say, ten one-minute intervals tell your rider that they can start from as little as 15 seconds, then 30, etc. Give them the permission. Make them aware they can stop any time they need.

You may wonder when to say these things. Ideally, before the class, but if you identify the issue during the class, switch the microphone off, walk over to that person and then say it.

Once you start the intervals, take time to walk over and stand next to them for maybe two intervals so they feel safe and push a bit harder as they know you are right next to them if anything happens.

Bring their attention to the breathing and the importance of recovery. There is also one super important point that we as seasoned instructors forget to mention – you know you do, too. The emergency break. We should mention it as a part of bike set up, but I guarantee you most of us don't. I make a point of showing this to this type of rider so they know even if I am not around and the fear takes over, they can make the pedals stop immediately.

A little one to one attention goes a long way and there is nothing more satisfactory than a rider who started like that who then builds confidence and starts pushing themselves until there comes a point that they just go solo and you no longer need to keep a close eye on them.

People Wearing Hoodies or Waist Trainers in Class

If you have seen any movies about people performing sports at high level, especially boxers, there is always a scene involving some hard-core workout while they wear numerous layers of clothing and a big hoodie on top. It is often done shortly before the weigh-in and a specific weight in sports like boxing or wrestling is of utmost importance as it determines your category.

I assume some people, entrepreneurs included, without the adequate knowledge of exercise science looked that that and thought: OK! So, to lose weight you must work hard while wearing loads of clothes which will make you sweat more. The more you sweat the more weight you lose. Bingo! Let me come up with an invention that will make people sweat more and then sell it as a weight loss enhancing thing.

The idea really took off in various forms. An example being studios who turn up the room temperature telling the riders they will work harder if they sweat more. I have already dealt with that myth in the chapter on Studio Temperature.

Every so often I will get a new rider come into the studio wearing a winter hoodie who is determined to keep it on. Thankfully I work on bikes with power meters and data, so I can show them the flaw in their philosophy in black and white *and* in colour using coach by colour system.

This simple and incorrect philosophy helped give birth to the special breed of leggings and underwear made of fabric that basically is totally non-breathable and so tight that putting these garments on is a workout in itself. If you think wearing them will significantly enhance your weight loss, think again.

The latest craze are the waist trainers. I like to call them wasters as their one and only contribution to your weight loss is a dent in your finances which you might have otherwise spent on food. Other than that, it's a waste of money.

To be fair, there is a statement on most of the websites selling these contraptions (which are not a new invention by all means but a modern version of a corset), saying that even though the waist trainer, 'will keep your abs tight and back straight and help you sweat extra during your workout,' which, 'may lead to quicker inch loss and weight loss,' one should **not** 'wear it while doing high intensity cardio or exercises that elevate your heart rate.'

That really made me laugh. Don't wear it during 'high intensity' exercise – understandable as it obstructs your breathing. Nor should you wear in doing exercise that 'elevates your heart rate'? Isn't that like *any* exercise? If you are doing an exercise that does not elevate your heart rate, is it even exercise?

Even if you think about easy yoga flows or gentle Pilates sequences, these focus on correct breathing which you cannot do while you are cinched at the waist. Therefore, the websites clearly state that while wearing the contraption *'may'* lead to quicker weight loss you should *not* wear it during any exercise.

Unfortunately, these days people do not read things carefully. We are bombarded with such an amount of information that all we do is skim a text and focus on what we want to see: 'quicker weight loss'.

There are many women, Kardashian followers or otherwise, who swear by these things. In my opinion these should not be called 'trainers' as they do not train anything. They are simply constrictors. If you wear this thing all day, or when you go out, you will automatically eat much less as your internal organs are so squashed you cannot overindulge, or you won't be able to breathe at all. That's all. And wearing them excessively or in wrong sizes can lead to deformation of internal organs as well as permanent changes to bone structures.

As far as cycling classes are concerned, if someone tells you they are wearing one of these or ask for your opinion, or if you simply notice someone wearing it, you should advise them to take it off for the class. I would even go as far as asking them to leave the studio if they refuse to take it off. If they insist on staying, let them but explain that if they feel dizzy, breathless or otherwise unwell once the intensity of the class increases, they had been warned.

www.ingramcontent.com/pod-product-compliance
Lightning Source LLC
LaVergne TN
LVHW051057080426
835508LV00019B/1931